Praise for
Gluten-Free on a Shoestring

"Hunn is clever and optimistic. As you flip through the pages, it's hard to avoid not feeling better about your gluten-free life. Plus, the recipes will inspire you to go into the kitchen with renewed energy and hope for the future. It's well worth spending money to purchase *Gluten-Free on a Shoestring*. It will pay dividends in the future."
—*Gluten-Free Living Magazine*

"Blogger-turned-cookbook author Hunn successfully tackles a chief complaint voiced by special-diet newbies: sticker shock. Her practical tips for shopping and cooking to save time and money are a gift to all of us who are paying too much for too little."
—*Living Without*

"Hunn has not only bestowed her readers with a complete cookbook . . . but she shows us how to save money, and time, on our meals. . . . It's well worth a bite."
—*San Francisco Book Review*

"[Hunn's] engaging writing style makes it seem like you have a good friend in the kitchen helping you along."
—*Gluten-Intolerance Group Magazine*

"It is the 125 recipes that make the book the most enjoyable, and if you are not part of the gluten-free world, then you may become a convert by book's end. . . . Get on the gluten-free bandwagon, finding ways to love these products, while at the same time creating recipes that are very friendly to the wallet."
—*Shelf Life*

Gluten-Free on a Shoestring

Quick and Easy

ALSO BY NICOLE HUNN

Gluten-Free on a Shoestring:
125 Easy Recipes for Eating Well on the Cheap (2011)

NICOLE HUNN

Gluten-Free on a
Shoestring
Quick and Easy

100 RECIPES FOR
THE FOOD YOU LOVE—FAST!

Da Capo
LIFE
LONG

*A Member of the
Perseus Books Group*

Set in 11 point Chaparral Pro by the Perseus Books Group

Cataloging-in-Publication data for this book is available from the Library of Congress.

First Da Capo Press edition 2012
ISBN 978-0-7382-1593-8 (paperback)
ISBN 978-0-7382-1609-6 (e-book)

Published by Da Capo Press
A Member of the Perseus Books Group
www.dacapopress.com

Da Capo Press books are available at special discounts for bulk purchases in the U.S. by corporations, institutions, and other organizations. For more information, please contact the Special Markets Department at the Perseus Books Group, 2300 Chestnut Street, Suite 200, Philadelphia, PA, 19103, or call (800) 810-4145, ext. 5000, or e-mail special.markets@perseusbooks.com.

10 9 8 7 6 5 4 3 2 1

To all my favorite children. You know who you are.

CONTENTS

4. Breads: Quicker and Quickest 53

5. Meatless Mondays
(or, Veggies Even My Pickiest Kid Might Eat) 87

8. Make-Your-Own Mixes
Pancake Mixes, Cake Mixes, Brownie Mixes, and More   189

INTRODUCTION

As a gluten-free food blogger and cookbook writer, I continue to be schooled—by you. I've learned so many things from reading and being read, writing and being written to.

Here's what I've learned: You're really busy.

Many of you are raising kids (often kids with special needs), and you don't have enough help. Or any help. You're trying to keep a career afloat, a house clean, and yourself and your family fed. You don't spend the same amount of time in the kitchen that I do, most days. You either don't want to, or can't, or a combination. Most important, you want, and deserve, plenty of food options.

I started out blogging at Gluten-Free on a Shoestring to let the gluten-free community in on what seemed like an open secret: Gluten-free food can be really expensive, but it doesn't always have to be. You don't have to buy a single frozen gluten-free muffin for $2.50. You can make your own muffin, and if you use an all-purpose gluten-free flour, the recipe can have seven ingredients, not twenty. And that muffin you make, it should taste as good as (if not better) than you remember, and it should (dare I say it) be readily affordable. It should make you proud and your non-gluten-free friends hungry. You don't have to buy frozen gluten-free dinners that cost seven dollars per person. You can make them better at home, and feed the whole family for about that same seven dollars. Gluten-free on the cheap was the goal of my first cookbook, *Gluten-Free on a Shoestring*. Mission accomplished. But now it's time to move on to . . . time.

This cookbook, *Gluten-Free on a Shoestring Quick and Easy*, is about shortcuts—saving you time and energy, *and* money. In this book, we'll tackle quick and delicious breakfasts for the weekday. As far as sandwiches go, you'll find some in-a-pinch quick breads that can hold up to sandwich fillings from chicken salad to nut butter and jelly. For those days when you have some more time to devote to bread baking, but still not as long as two hours, there are quick-rise yeast bread recipes inside, as well as refrigerator dough that you can let rise on the weekend, and then bake as you need all week long. And because weekdays can be hectic but you still gotta eat, there are enough budget- and time-conscious dinners—some with meat, some without—to please everyone. For the big finish, we have some quick cakes and pies, plus lots of make-your-own mixes for everything from cookies and muffins to cakes and pancakes. Plus my pitch for why a make-your-own mix is both a smart move and easy to do.

Since the first *Shoestring* came out, so much has happened in the gluten-free community. The landscape has changed forever and for the better. Gluten-free is now chic. Have you heard? We've gone all Hollywood and stuff, and all the glitterati are eating gluten-free just for the heck of it, or the general health benefits. Other than the fact that I now always make sure I wear clean clothes while cooking (one can never predict with true accuracy the next photo-op), what does this new-found status really mean for us?

Good things. First, there are now more and better gluten-free packaged food options than I could have ever dreamed possible even two years ago. When I wrote *Gluten-Free on a Shoestring*, baking with an all-purpose gluten-free flour such as Better Batter, rather than with several single-component gluten-free flours, seemed revolutionary. Today, an all-purpose substitute is commonplace (and for good reason). Plus, gluten-free packaged bread is now more widely available, and it is priced more reasonably (and, although it still has a ways to go, believe you me—it's going). Such increased options and availability usually mean lower prices and higher quality. Case in point: Kellogg's introduction of a gluten-free reformulation of Rice Krispies, sold at the same price as its conventional counterpart. Score one for Team Gluten Free.

It works roughly like this: Gluten-free food manufacturers now have the economies of scale they needed to bring their costs down (because the more a producer buys from suppliers, the more leverage that producer has in negotiating prices). What's more, when these food manufacturers can sell more of those gluten-free products, they can lower their profit margins and still do a very good business, thank you very much. Then, the food manufacturers that can't (or simply won't) provide us with the quality we deserve, and the price we are increasingly able to demand, go out of business. Then more competitive businesses take their place. Capitalism. A beautiful thing sometimes.

Second, there's more, credible information about celiac disease and gluten intolerance and sensitivity out there than ever before—and it's more accessible. We are such a motivated and growing community, and so very chic, that some of the biggest food manufacturers in the country (such as General Mills) are taking notice. They're redoubling their efforts, not only to provide gluten-free prepared foods, but also to serve the needs of the gluten-free community with such information resources as GlutenFreely.com. They're telling us that their commitment to us is real. Do I hear wedding bells?

Finally, now that our basic needs are being met, we have the luxury of expecting more convenient, inexpensive gluten-free meals. Enter *Gluten-Free on a Shoestring, Quick and Easy*. We can, and should, now be able to put together a family meal in about half an hour. We can buy conventional corn tortillas, many of which are now proudly labeled gluten-free, and press them into service for dinner in a flash. How about a quick stir-fry using Annie Chun's Rice Noodles, with a cheeky "Gluten Free" badge right on the package? We can buy cake mixes to ensure consistently reliable results in a pinch—and even make our own mixes almost as easily ("Mom! There's a birthday party tomorrow in school!"). Don't want to buy any convenience products, but still want good food fast? I've got you completely covered with tons of other shortcuts (such as yeast-free gluten-free bread!) to keep that kitchen of yours humming along.

With this book, we'll be together every step of the way, taking convenient shortcuts to amazing gluten-free meals the whole family will love. It's high time to take it easy.

And remember—life is sweet and fun. As always, gluten is expendable.

....

Chapter 1

Low-Down, Dirty, Quick, and Easy Basics

Whenever I cook at home, I aim for a gluten-free meal that every member of the family can get behind in a big way, all on a shoestring budget. The food has to be unfussy, because I'm a home cook and I don't like to fuss. I'll leave the fuss to restaurant chefs. I've always sought hearty dishes that satisfy both body and soul, as food is one of life's great pleasures. If you know me at all, that should come as no surprise.

Now, it's time for a new chapter. In *Gluten-Free on a Shoestring, Quick and Easy*, as with my first cookbook, you'll still find good, solid family food that is reliably gluten-free and won't break the bank. But this time, we pick up the pace.

I recognize that not everyone has a lot of time to spend in the kitchen. Nor should you be expected to. Maybe your yoga instructor spends her free time trying to learn to spin like a top on the crown of her head. That doesn't mean that even the most advanced students should strive for the same in their off hours. So this time I have that idea top of mind as we get moving.

I've bought us some time with the mad multitasking skills that I'll teach you to put to use in the kitchen. You'll learn to master recipes that make use of both fast-acting ingredients in place of slower-acting ones and the most worthwhile store-bought gluten-free ingredients to augment a meal. And there are even a few new pieces of fast-paced kitchen equipment that might earn a place on your counter.

Time

There's no shortage of clichés about time, but one thing's for certain. Time is the one resource we can never renew. On a busy weekday evening when everyone's hungry, we don't usually find ourselves with time to kill. We want fast prep, quick cooking times, and minimal cleanup. And we don't want to compromise on taste or nutrition to get it.

In these recipes, part of the time is reclaimed through good, old-fashioned shortcut methods such as substituting slower ingredients like yeast with faster ones like baking powder (or by taking advantage of a slow second rise for yeast in the refrigerator during the week). As I began recipe development, I realized that I was gravitating toward speedier versions of many of the recipes that I had been making for years. I was pleasantly surprised when I realized that I could make good gluten-free and yeast-free English muffins (page XXX) without sacrificing taste. And they're ready quickly enough to have for a weeknight meal—made from scratch that very night! After some trial and error, I found that I could make a yeast-free sandwich bread as well. That meant it could be ready as fast as any other quick bread, with such leaveners as baking powder and baking soda, and a few other stabilizing ingredients.

Most of the recipes in this cookbook take less than forty minutes to prepare, and the few that take a bit longer either have portions that can and should be made in advance or the remaining time is inactive. Every recipe you'll find here, from the yeast-free doughnuts (pages 42 and 44) to the Quick Puff Pastry (page 82), is quicker and easier than its original version. The doughnuts come together more like muffins, without yeast, and are ready quickly, especially in the four-minute cycle of a Babycakes Mini Donut Maker. The Quick Puff Pastry is, indeed, speedy, but keep in mind that there's no way to make any sort of puff pastry without doing some "turns." Making black beans from scratch is always going to be slower than opening a can of cooked black beans. But the Pressure Cooker Scratch Black Beans (page 96) take about forty minutes from start to finish, and that's if you haven't presoaked the beans. If you have, it takes even less time. Either way, the quality and cost is far superior to canned beans, making the beans more versatile and more useful.

Throughout the book, I also provide time-saving tips such as using unbleached parchment paper for rolling out dough with a French rolling pin (the kind without handles that is tapered on both ends). Those two tweaks alone can shave ten to fifteen minutes off your active cooking time, not to mention increasing your success rate. But you have to absorb the tips, and collect the supplies. Then try it yourself, in your own kitchen.

Working quickly in the kitchen requires multitasking, even if it's for a one-pot dinner. While water is boiling, onions are being chopped. While onions are cooking, vegetables are being chopped. The recipe instructions are written to make the most of the time you do spend in the kitchen, so you can sit down to eat faster. It's like learning a dance. The more you practice, the more muscle memory you have for the steps.

Some of the weeknight meals take advantage of store-bought gluten-free convenience foods. They can be a tremendous help on a night when you just don't feel like making bread from scratch, even if you now know how to bake some fresh in twenty minutes flat. My general rule of thumb is that if the bread is central to the meal, such as a veggie burger on an English muffin (see Yeast-Free English Muffins, page 55), I'll make the muffin from scratch. If not, I won't.

Sometimes, instead of quicker "from scratch" food, the solution is the smart use of make-ahead recipes. For example, I found that the very same dough from the White Sandwich Bread recipe in my first cookbook would keep in the refrigerator for days, its flavor only becoming more complex and savory day after day. That meant that a fresh batch of even yeasted rolls could be made on a weeknight. I've included that recipe here as a bonus, along with the recipe from my first book for Flour Tortillas (page 80). Their versatility can't be beat.

Kitchen Confidence

A word about recipe cooking times and what I call "kitchen confidence": the time estimate that is indicated in the recipes is just that, an estimate. It assumes some basic cooking fluency. The truth is that practice makes perfect. If you've never rolled out pizza dough before, it's not going to take you less than ten minutes to roll out two pies. No matter how well written a recipe is, there is no substitute for actually trying your own hand at it.

If you're not as confident cooking gluten-free as you'd like to be (like I once was—I cried the first time I tried to bake gluten-free bread), know that you can, indeed, feed yourself and your family well, on time, and on budget. Gluten-free cooking and baking should not be precious or out of reach. Today, they're safely within *your* reach. In fact, it's easier than ever to get the job done. But you have to practice. If you'd like to become proficient at rolling out pizza dough, set aside a stress-free thirty minutes on a weekend to learn about it. Read through the recipe for Refrigerator Pizza Dough White Pizza (page 106) a few times. Take out all of your ingredients, just as the recipe describes. Do it methodically, without deviating from the recipe if possible.

The more you practice, the faster you'll get. You may even find yourself beating the time estimate, putting me to shame! Master a few signature dishes or desserts. Then place those in your weekday rotation, and don't be afraid to repeat the same dish a couple of times in one week. Once you begin to feel more confident and have some time to spare, try something new. Maybe you've got a random day off scheduled from work, just to use up some vacation time. Why not schedule a solitary cooking and baking session for yourself? First, page through this book chapter by chapter, a cup of coffee in hand. Select one or two dishes that you'd like to eat if someone else prepared them for you. Make a shopping list, and go shop it. Come back, lay out, and prep all the ingredients. Reread the ingredients and instructions one last time, and then get to work. There's plenty of time to customize the recipe later once you've mastered it as written. You'll get there, step by step.

Convenience Pantry Items to Buy

All of the recipes in this book are meant to be as user-friendly as possible. Every ingredient, with a few notable exceptions such as good all-purpose gluten-free flour (see page 9), is either available in a large local supermarket or can be replaced by one that is. You won't find any hard-to-find or hard-to-pronounce ingredients here.

These recipes evolved as my thinking did. For years, there had been ready-made gluten-free products available for purchase. But most of them had to be mail-ordered, the prices were outrageously high, and the quality was often lacking. That led many to judge gluten-free packaged goods by the "it's good—for gluten-free" standard. In my last cookbook, I railed against the low standards many in the gluten-free community had been conditioned to have. Demand more and the market will bear it!

Well, we did. And it has. There's still some ways to go (will some large food manufacturer please put out ready-made gluten-free wonton skins?) but convenience foods are getting there. Now we can make use of the growing number of high-quality packaged gluten-free products—and open a package of cookies or bread just as our gluten-eating friends and neighbors can.

Here are a few of my favorite gluten-free convenience food items, many of which you'll see scattered through the recipes in this book. Don't worry—the cost still won't even compare to complete ready-made meals, either from the frozen foods section or from a gluten-free restaurant. Or to those "it's good—for gluten-free" packaged cookies and muffins:

- **Idaho Spuds Brand Signature Potato Bits:** Try them and you'll know why these really are that much better than other brands. I'm all for real potatoes, but that doesn't mean I don't know how to appreciate a good bud or bit when I see one.

- **Gluten-free packaged corn tortillas:** Because a flexible and tasty gluten-free flour tortilla is not widely available just yet, I am grateful to have packaged corn tortillas available. Just be sure to read labels to make sure that your brand is, in fact, gluten-free (Del Campo brand soft corn tortillas are gluten-free, as of the writing of this book). When you warm them up either in the microwave wrapped in a wet paper towel or in a skillet right before you sit down to eat, they taste nearly fresh.

- **Shredded cheeses:** I buy blocks of cheese, but I also buy bags of already shredded cheeses. They tend to be a bit dry as compared to freshly grated cheese, so I use them in places where that doesn't matter—such as on pizza. I always grate Parmigiano-Reggiano fresh with a Microplane, but I don't always grate mozzarella cheese fresh. Now you know. Judge me accordingly. Oh, and do buy blocks of real Parmigiano-Reggiano. It has so much flavor, it could power a jet, if flavor powered jets. A little really does go a long way, and save the rinds for flavoring soups and sauces.

- **Gluten-free rotisserie chicken:** These days, warehouse stores such as Costco and even many major supermarkets sell cooked rotisserie chickens that are reliably gluten-free. It's so nice to buy one and just build an easy meal around it. I don't do it every week, but I absolutely don't hesitate to buy one when I know it's going to be a hectic week.

- **Sliced sandwich bread, such as Udi's or Rudi's:** Gluten-free packaged sliced sandwich breads are growing in number, and my local Trader Joe's even sells Udi's bread unfrozen. Glory be! It's not even frozen! And they sell out of it nearly every day. But I've come to realize that it's nice to have a loaf of Udi's or Rudi's in my freezer for my kids' school lunches. Sometimes, there are big air pockets in a loaf and I get on my high horse and promise never to buy it again. And then I buy it again. I hope it gets better and less expensive, but I'm still glad to have a stash.

- **Schär Parbaked Ciabatta and French Breads:** These parbaked breads are vacuum-sealed, so they tend to have a nice, luxuriously long shelf life. Oh how I love it when foods are vacuum-sealed! My general rule of thumb is that, when the meal is built around the bread you are serving, make it from scratch whenever possible. Otherwise, and if you're pressed for time, all you do is peel open the bag of Schär parbaked bread, pop it in the toaster oven or conventional oven for about ten minutes, and voilà! Fresh-tasting bread. It's rather expensive, but I like having it around. It's like a dinnertime security blanket. Hold me?

- **Gluten-free chicken and vegetable stock:** In *Gluten-Free on a Shoestring*, I was the queen of make-your-own-stock. And I still do make my own. Long live the queen! But more often than not these days, I find myself willing to renounce the throne. Pacific Natural Foods chicken and vegetable stocks are reliably gluten-free, often on sale or special, and just plain taste good. I never really buy beef stock. If I am making beef, it makes its own stock and I'd rather cook with something a bit lighter that doesn't overpower the other flavors in the dish.

❧ **No-stir nut butters:** I really like Barney Butter smooth almond butter and Peanut Butter & Co. Smooth Operator peanut butter. Barney Butter is mondo expensive, though, and never really seems to go on sale. Peanut Butter & Co. is relatively affordable, and it's just so good. No-stir nut butters relieve me of the burden (yes, I did just say burden, and I don't consider it melodramatic) of having to bend multiple spoons trying to stir down a traditional natural nut butter. And I find that, no matter how much elbow grease I put into it, there is still a completely oil-free nut butter rock at the bottom of the jar. I also learned that when you buy a thick nut butter, it is easy to spread a satisfying layer of the stuff on bread without globbing the whole jar onto a sandwich. And these consistently smooth nut butters are great for cooking and baking. Okay, I'll stop now. I've gone on long enough about nut butters. Unless you want to know more . . .

❧ **Triple-washed, bagged fresh baby spinach:** I've moved past frozen spinach. I have. I buy the triple-washed stuff. I put it in everything these days. I don't have to defrost it, I don't have to squeeze it (I hate squeezing water out of vegetables; see potato bits missive earlier), and it's so easy to wilt. And you know what? They wash it for you three whole times, but they don't charge that much for it. Gosh, I hope they have good labor practices.

❧ **Good tomato sauce:** Add tomato sauce to anything and you give it an instant hit of flavor, and usually some extra body and texture, too. When I'm making the One-Pot Albondigas Dinner (page 117), I'm not going to be bothered making my own tomato sauce to thicken that broth. How would that be quick and easy? Get something pretty good, too—nothing that tastes like it's a few paces away from passing as ketchup, please. It doesn't have to be the best for eight dollars a jar, but if you look for it, you can find a 25-ounce jar of Muir Glen tomato sauce for not much more than three dollars. It's worth it.

❧ **Breakfast cereal for use as "bread" crumbs:** I buy a few boxes of gluten-free breakfast cereals such as gluten-free Chex and gluten-free Erewhon crisp rice–style cereals when they're on sale, and I get to work. I process them in my food processor, store them in a resealable container in my pantry, and I never want for bread crumbs. I really don't enjoy washing and drying my food processor, so I make a bunch at a time. If you enjoy such things, I'll give you 5 bucks to wash and dry mine.

- **Schär shortbread-style and other cookies, for a great cheesecake crust when ground:** Here I go, Schär-ing again. But I really do like them. Their products are a bit spendy sometimes, but I don't buy these things all the time. When I do, I want them to be top-notch. These cookies taste really good, and believe it or not there are times when I don't have any homemade gluten-free cookies lying around. Okay, it doesn't happen much since I bake pathologically at this point, but it does happen. And when it does, I like to have Schär short-bread cookies in my pantry. They make an excellent No-Bake Cheesecake (page 166) crust, and sign up for the Schär Club (www.schar.com/us/club -benefits/) to find coupons to make them more shoestring-friendly.

Last but not least, the most important convenience item I have in my pantry is my all-purpose gluten-free flour blend.

A NOTE ABOUT GLUTEN-FREE FLOURS

Better Batter All Purpose Gluten Free Flour

The recipes in this cookbook that incorporate flour call for an all-purpose gluten-free flour blend. My favorite, based on basic quality and price criteria, is made by Better Batter Gluten Free Flour. It's a high-quality premade flour blend containing rice flour, brown rice flour, tapioca starch, potato starch, potato flour, xanthan gum, and pectin (a lemon derivative). It's a proprietary formula, and I know nothing of the proportions. So when Better Batter runs out of flour, so do I. And this whole operation is in shambles! That's why I buy it in bulk.

Better Batter is as true a replacement for conventional, gluten-containing all-purpose flour as I have found. It has a very fine grain, and to me tastes "normal." I have used it successfully for years, in everything from yeast breads and doughnuts to muffins and cakes. It does behave a bit differently than its conventional, gluten-containing counterpart, but that is to be expected. Gluten is such an essential component of conventional flour that it's difficult for me to imagine anyone creating a gluten-free blend that truly mimics gluten in every conceivable way without alteration, including in yeast breads. I've found that this one is close enough.

That said, many companies these days make all-purpose gluten-free flours. Perhaps your personal experience has been different and you have found another commercially available gluten-free flour blend that suits all of your needs. Or maybe you have perfected your own blend of gluten-free component flours in proportions that make it all-purpose. I strongly encourage you to use your preferred high-quality blend in any of my recipes that call for all-purpose gluten-free flour. My only suggestion is that you measure your blend by weight, and not by volume, to ensure an accurate measurement. Different gluten-free flours, and therefore different gluten-free flour blends, have different weights by volume.

Other Premade All-Purpose Gluten-Free Flours

In addition to Better Batter, I have tested extensively three other commercially available gluten-free flour blends—Cup4Cup Gluten Free Flour, Tom Sawyer Gluten Free Flour, and Jules Gluten Free All Purpose Flour—in various categories of recipes, and scored for those blends along with Better Batter in ten separate ratings categories. I recorded the results on my blog. If you are trying to decide which premade blend is best for you, those results are worth a look here: http://glutenfreeonashoestring.com/the-great-gluten-free-flour-test/.

Please note that bean flour blends that are marketed as "all-purpose gluten-free flour" are not even close to being appropriate for all purposes. They behave *very* differently from the high-quality blends discussed here, and will not work in my recipes. The same is true for multi-ingredient baking mixes, such as Pamela's Baking Mix and Bisquick Gluten Free, which are not intended to be used as all-purpose gluten-free flours, as they contain ingredients such as baking powder, baking soda, and salt.

Do-It-Yourself All-Purpose Gluten-Free Flour

If you would like to blend your own all-purpose gluten-free flour, I have tested a DIY blend that I can now recommend, and which follows. I have not tried it in every single one of my recipes, either on the blog or in my cookbooks, but I have tried it in every recipe category and found its performance to be comparable to that of Better Batter.

A few words of caution: To consider this blend a high-quality gluten-free flour blend that is good for all baking purposes, you *must* use superfine rice flours and all of your components must be high quality and certified gluten-free. The only source in the United States for these flours I am aware of is Authentic Foods (http://authenticfoods.com/). And Authentic Foods superfine flours do not come particularly cheap. You may be able to find component flours at your local ethnic market, but there are myriad possibilities of cross-contamination with gluten both in manufacturing, in transit, and even in the store itself. Please also note that, when done right, this blend is nearly twice as expensive per cup as Better Batter (please see my blog for detailed cost analyses of all these blends). And the ingredients are not sold in packages that correspond to the proportions in which you need them in the blend. You will alternate between too much rice flour and too much starch, creating a round robin of ingredient purchases.

Here is my DIY all-purpose gluten-free flour blend. The recipe can be quartered, halved, doubled, tripled, quadrupled, etc., at will:

160 grams superfine brown rice flour from Authentic Foods
160 grams superfine white rice flour from Authentic Foods
 80 grams tapioca starch/flour from Authentic Foods
 80 grams potato starch from Authentic Foods
 20 grams potato flour from Authentic Foods
 18 grams high-quality xanthan gum from Bob's Red Mill
  8 grams pure powdered fruit pectin from Pomona Pectin
    (http://www.pomonapectin.com)

Simply place all of these ingredients in a large, airtight container, and whisk well. Secure the container closed until ready to use. The blend will be as shelf stable as its component flours. To extend the shelf life, store the container in the refrigerator or freezer.

Individual Gluten-Free Flours

There are probably as many ways to assemble various gluten-free flours—such as rice flour, sorghum flour, and almond flour—into various blends as there are stars in the sky. Some may work extremely well in cakes, others in yeast breads. Some may make the flakiest pastries you think you've ever tasted, and others the best roux for your grandmother's gumbo. I bought many component gluten-free flours in 2004 when I started baking gluten-free. I panicked. A lot. I cried, probably as often. There was little guidance available at the time, and I craved simplicity at least as much as I craved a good doughnut. As soon as I found a good all-purpose blend, I felt a tremendous sense of relief. I could leave the food science largely to the flour-making people, and do the rest myself. I now have the DIY flour blend I spoke about earlier, but I don't use it regularly. I use Better Batter day in and day out. I've also found finely ground almond flour to be useful as a dairy-free protein substitute for whey powder (see Dairy-Free Make-Your-Own Vanilla Cake Mix, page 195).

In the name of progress, I have also begun to experiment with adding whole-grain gluten-free flours to some of my gluten-free recipes. It's like in your pre-gluten-free days, using conventional all-purpose white flour, and then moving on to adding some whole wheat flour, followed by a bit of rye flour if you were feeling adventurous. I find that I enjoy working with whole-grain teff, a gluten-free supergrain. Stabilized rice bran also adds quite a lot of nutrients and fiber, and a heartiness that I like. But those recipes are not the subject of this book. Some of those recipes have found their way onto my blog. More will follow. I promise not to deprive you of any of them.

Gluten-Free on a Shoestring, Quick and Easy means just that. Always affordable, and now quick and easy, too. I find that mixing component gluten-free flours into different blends is neither quick, nor easy. Plus, as discussed earlier, it's not usually very cost effective, either. For this book, I stick with straight up, high-quality all-purpose gluten-free flour—however you define that. If you have a history with your own blend of flours, or another commercially prepared blend that suits all of your needs, by all means, feel free to use it gram for gram wherever a recipe calls for a high-quality all-purpose gluten-free flour.

In the next chapter, we'll talk about the equipment and tools that help you make good food fast. They really are worth rearranging your kitchen cabinets to find a bit of space to store them.

Chapter 2

....

Make-It-Snappy Kitchen Tools and Equipment

We've talked about time, that jealous mistress, and how we can bend it to meet our needs. Now let's run down the tools and equipment that can really help make quick work of food prep, cooking, and storage. You can get by without many of these products, but each of them has become indispensable in my kitchen for helping me move fast when it matters most. Every one is affordable on most budgets, and you don't need to acquire them all at once. I'll tell you about why I love each of them. Then, you decide.

8-quart pressure cooker: If you're afraid of pressure cookers because you think they have a tendency to explode in one's face, fear no more. Today's pressure cookers are smart. If too much pressure builds up in one of the modern-day pressure cookers, they simply let off just enough steam to equalize it. (I can totally relate.) To use these smart pressure cookers, all you do is add your ingredients, secure the lid, and bring the pot to pressure over medium-high heat. You'll know that it's reached pressure when the little button on the handle pops. And no, you don't have to stare at the button (a watched button never pops anyway, right?). It pops audibly. Usually, I'm reading the newspaper and I jump when it pops (using a pressure cooker means I get to read the paper). Then, start your timer. When the specified time has elapsed, either let the pressure reduce naturally once you remove the pot from the heat, or run cold water over the top of the pot, which will reduce the pressure quickly. Then, you can safely remove the lid and enjoy.

I have the Fagor Duo 8-quart pressure cooker. I bought mine right off the shelf at Bed Bath & Beyond, and I used a Shoestring-friendly 20 percent coupon (don't have one? I'll send you one), and it ended up costing me less than eighty dollars. It's simple to use and comes with a booklet that has some sample recipe ideas and cooking times. At 8 quarts, it isn't too big to store in my cabinets, but it has sufficient capacity for anything I want to make for my family of five. My pressure cooker also reaches a high pressure of 15 psi, which cooks food significantly faster than one that only reaches 8 psi. Be sure yours reaches 15 psi.

Babycakes Mini Doughnut Maker: I can't even believe I'm including this ridiculous machine in this roundup. But I can't help myself. I love this little electric doughnut maker. I actually find this machine easier to store than a doughnut pan, which is more unwieldy in size and shape. This little machine is compact, and although it only makes six mini doughnuts at a time, one cycle is only four minutes. Four minutes from batter to hot doughnut! And I have two doughnut recipes that are perfectly suited to this bad boy: Yeast-Free Glazed Plain Doughnuts (page 42) and Yeast-Free Glazed Chocolate Doughnuts (page 44). When you make doughnuts in a doughnut pan, it can be tough to get them to be evenly domed on the top. Not so with this little machine. You know you want one. Just promise me you won't buy the Whoopie Pie Maker? Unless you do, and you love it, and think I should get one. And then tell me and I'll think about it. Never say never.

Immersion blender: Ever try to blend soup in a blender? How about a smoothie in a blender? I don't care how careful you are, it makes a mess. Enter the immersion blender, also known as a stick blender. The bottom part detaches from the base, so cleanup couldn't be easier. When I'm making Vegetarian Chili (page 112), I like to blend some of it before serving so that it's thicker. It tastes better to me, and it makes it easier for my kids to eat it. Thank you, immersion blender!

Tortilla press and tortilla warmer: I have a cast-aluminum tortilla press. It's nothing fancy, but it helps get my Flour Tortillas (page 80) started in the right direction. I still roll them out, but when they get a head start in the press, it's so much easier for me to get a rhythm going. I press, roll, sear in the hot pan. Press, roll, sear. And then I put the hot tortillas, one right on top of the other, in my tortilla warmer. That's not fancy, either—it's really just a round plastic container with a lid—but it keeps the tortillas warm and moist for hours until I'm ready to use them. All I do is place a wet paper towel on the bottom of the warmer before I place the first tortilla inside. And then, once I've made all the tortillas, I flip over the stack so the bottom tortilla becomes the top tortilla. That way, none of them gets soggy. I have the Vasconia aluminum 7½-inch tortilla press, and the Imusa tortilla warmer.

Digital kitchen scale: Wherever possible, the recipes in this book contain both volume and weight measurements. But I'm secretly hoping that you'll use the weight measurements. A kitchen scale makes really quick work of measuring dry ingredients, as you just keep putting dry ingredients into one bowl, zeroing out the weight after each addition by pushing the Tare button (yup; that's what that button is for). It is also the only truly precise way to measure dry ingredients that are present in any sizable quantity.

When I measure Better Batter all-purpose gluten-free flour, my "cup" is 140 grams, so that is my benchmark. If you are using your own blend of flours, or any blend, for that matter, it is particularly important that you measure by weight. The flour that you are using could be much denser than Better Batter, making a volume measurement all but irrelevant. My digital scale is inexpensive, and I haven't broken it yet. It's an Escali Primo multifunctional digital scale. Don't be fooled by the word *primo*. It could just as easily be named *básico*. And it's, frankly, *perfecto*.

Seasoned cast-iron pans: I have only one omelet pan, and it is the only nonstick skillet I own. Nonstick coatings degrade over time to the point where every supposed nonstick pan I had was becoming decidedly "stick." I haven't yet found a reasonable replacement for the nonstick omelet pan, but for everything else I use seasoned cast-iron skillets. They conduct and retain heat so well that your food cooks quickly and evenly. For everything from shallow frying to cooking Flour Tortillas (page 80), my Lodge seasoned cast-iron skillet and griddle are unequaled.

USA Pan bakeware: If you've been to my blog, you know how I love USA Pan. It's a family-owned company, it makes all its products in the good old US of A, and it offers heirloom quality products at eminently reasonable prices.

USA Pan bakeware is the only nonstick bakeware I'll use. It's made nonstick by baking the same material as you'll find in a Silpat nonstick baking liner right onto the pan. So nothing sticks to it, but, unlike Teflon, it lasts forever because it doesn't degrade from use. It also doesn't make you sick or warp in the oven. USA's 8½ by 4½-inch loaf pan is the best loaf pan I have ever used, bar none. I've had mine for three years, and still don't grease it. My bread just pops right out when I tip the pan. It's that easy. I also really love my USA Pan small Pullman loaf pan, which I use without the cover. And food bakes so evenly because of both the quality of the materials, and the raised striations on the surface, which allow air to circulate. They are truly a must-have for the gluten-free baker.

The company has been around for many years, but only in the last few years has it been in the retail business. Before that, it only sold to wholesalers, and it makes many of the upscale house-brand baking sheets that you've seen in Williams-Sonoma and Sur La Table. Ooh-la-la at a *yawn* price.

Unbleached parchment paper: In *Gluten-Free on a Shoestring*, we were busy rolling out all of our gluten-free dough with plastic wrap. Bleached parchment paper was too stiff and thick, making it impossible to feel the dough under the paper. Enter unbleached parchment paper. It's much thinner and more flexible than the bleached kind, and it doesn't burn. If You Care is an excellent brand. If you can get past feeling judged by the name, you'll be using this stuff a whole lot. And it's environmentally conscious. Turns out, I do care!

French rolling pin: A French rolling pin is the kind that is tapered on both ends and doesn't have any handles. I have one made by Ateco. It makes a huge difference in one's ability to roll out gluten-free dough (with that parchment paper we talked about), because you can control where you place the pressure and how much pressure you use on the dough—two very important features in dough rolling.

Extra measuring spoons: Why did it take me so long to realize that it would be so much easier if I had just one more set of measuring spoons? Certain ingredients, such as salt and yeast when making bread, really should not be commingled. If you use the same measuring spoon in your salt, and then dip it into your yeast, you could kill the yeast. Dead. This is life or death, people.

Ateco cookie cutter sets: I have a set of concentric circle cookie cutters. They come in handy all the time. Rather than trying to collect all the right sizes of cutters, I bought the whole set at once. They're very good quality, so they don't rust or warp, and they come in a neat little tin, which is important if you're anything like me and have no idea how to store cookie cutters otherwise.

Small offset spatula: I use this angled spatula for everything from spreading frosting on a cake to lifting something delicate from counter to baking sheet. It's so comfortable, it feels like an extension of my hand. My 9-inch offset (also called angled) spatula is made by Wilton, and has a nicely curved black handle.

Balloon whisk: When a recipe's instructions call for whisking together dry ingredients, it really and truly does matter whether you follow the instructions. Leaveners such as baking powder and baking soda have to be evenly distributed throughout the dough to work, or some portions of your baked goods will rise too much and others not at all. Please practice safe baking. Whisk.

Flat whisk: A balloon whisk is great for dry ingredients in a bowl, but it can be maddening to try to use it to get into the corners of saucepans. A flat whisk is made for that purpose. You won't use it as often as you use the balloon whisk, but you'll be so happy to have it when you need it.

Bench scraper: There's nothing like a floured bench scraper (originally the sole province of construction workers) to divide dough into portions.

Freezer-safe bags and wraps: I am asked often about how to store gluten-free bread. Yeast bread dough should not be frozen raw, but once baked, the bread freezes quite well. However, nothing freezes well if it is ravaged by freezer burn. Since I am unwilling to invest both money and counter space in a vacuum sealer (not to mention the fact that I'm terrified that I'd melt my own self in that hot thing), I use Ziploc freezer safe storage bags and Glad Press'n Seal for the freezer.

Bread bin: For keeping home-baked bread fresh, if you can spare the counter space, a bread bin is very nice. It allows you to slice what you need from a fresh loaf of bread and then return it to the bread bin without wrapping it in plastic. The loaf will still be fresh when you are ready to slice it again. It's staggering how expensive some wooden bread bins are—enough to tempt me right into a new woodworking hobby. Instead, I bought a retro-looking metal Polder bin on Amazon.com. Cheaper than a new hobby, I think.

You do also need a sharp chef's knife or Japanese ***santoku*** (I have a Wusthof brand *santoku*), and I find that I move so much faster when I keep my knife sharp. Except when it's too sharp, because of the first aid that sometimes has to be administered, which tends to slow a cook down like nobody's business.

All in all, you don't need a whole lot to move quickly in your kitchen. So, let's get cooking and baking. On your mark, get set. . . . Go!

Chapter 3

Breakfast and Brunch

I n the world of food and nutrition, we're given so many mixed and changing messages: Don't eat any fat. Eat only fat. Eat mostly meat. No, no, just eat vegetables. Eat like a caveman. Eat local.

I try not to get too involved.

But there is one piece of advice that hasn't changed since, well, forever, and I feel pretty safe living by it: Eat breakfast. Whoever you are, whatever you do all day, you want to get yourself moving with some high-quality protein. I'm a big fan of eggs, but they're not always practical when the school bus leaves at 7:30 a.m. That's where the homemade protein bars and granola cookies in this chapter come in. They keep for a long while in the refrigerator, and they also freeze well. Some version of them is always resident in my refrigerator, and everyone in the family loves them.

Also in this chapter: weekend goodies that will have the whole family lingering at the table. Try the yeast-free doughnuts that are ready in mere minutes. The savory breakfast polenta, Texas Toast, mini potato quiches, and baked oatmeal round out the offerings.

- ✿ Quick Potato Crust Quiche
- ✿ Quicker, Dairy-Free Cinnamon Buns
- ✿ Quickest, Yeast-Free Cinnamon Buns

- No-Bake Berry Breakfast Protein Bars
- No-Bake Chocolate Breakfast Protein Bars
- Vegan Granola Protein Bites
- Pumpkin Granola Breakfast Cookies
- Chocolate Popovers
- Egg in the Hole
- German Pancake
- Chocolate Breakfast Muffins
- Yeast-Free Glazed Plain Doughnuts
- Yeast-Free Glazed Chocolate Doughnuts
- Breakfast Burritos
- Texas Toast
- Muesli
- Morning Polenta
- Baked Oatmeal
- Drop Biscuits

Quick Potato Crust Quiche

Time Estimate: 15 minutes active time, 30 minutes inactive time

MAKES 4 SERVINGS

Can be doubled to make 2 quiches easily

I've made some relatively complicated quiches in my time. They were nice. I was tired. I've also made some super simple, down-and-dirty no-crust quiches. Some of the members of my household were not amused. This little number is the best of both worlds. It doesn't involve peeling or grating (the work! the squeezing!) or even boiling potatoes, but it still has a potato crust. How can it be? One word (okay, five): Idaho Spuds Signature Potato Bits.

½ cup (35g) Idaho Spuds brand Signature Potato Bits

½ to ¾ cup (70 to 105 g) high-quality all-purpose gluten-free flour

¼ teaspoon xanthan gum (omit if your blend already contains it)

½ teaspoon kosher salt

5 tablespoons (70 g) roughly chopped and chilled unsalted butter

¼ to ½ cup water, iced (cubes don't count in the volume measurement)

6 extra-large eggs, at room temperature, beaten

½ cup milk (the richer the milk, the richer the quiche)

4 ounces shredded Cheddar cheese

½ teaspoon freshly ground black pepper, or to taste

10 ounces frozen broccoli, thawed, drained, and chopped

1. In the bowl of your food processor fitted with the metal blade, place the potato bits, ½ cup (70 g) of the flour, the xanthan gum, and ¼ teaspoon of salt, and pulse until well mixed. Add the cold, chopped butter and pulse a few times. The mixture should be relatively dry. If it seems too moist, as if it might just hold together already, add the remaining ¼ cup (35 g) of flour a tablespoon at a time, and pulse to mix.

2. Add ¼ cup of ice-cold water by the tablespoon to the mixture and pulse to mix. The dough should begin to come together. If much of it is still not holding together, add more water by the tablespoon until it just begins to form a ball.

3. Turn out the dough onto a piece of plastic wrap, wrap tightly, and place in the freezer to firm while you make the quiche filling.

4. Preheat your oven to 375°F. Grease a standard 9-inch pie plate with unsalted butter and set it aside.

5. In a large bowl, whisk together the eggs, milk, cheese, remaining ¼ teaspoon of salt and the pepper. Add the broccoli, and mix well. Set the mixture aside.

6. Remove the dough from the freezer and unwrap the plastic wrap. Place the dough between two sheets of unbleached parchment paper, and roll into a round about 6 inches in diameter. Place the round in the center of the prepared pie plate, and press into the edges and up the sides as evenly as you can. Pour the quiche filling into the center of the pie plate.

7. Bake the quiche in the center of the oven for 30 minutes, or until set and golden around the edges. Allow to cool slightly, then slice and serve.

Shoestring Savings

On a shoestring: $1.20/serving

If you bought it: $3.47/serving

Quicker, Dairy-Free Cinnamon Buns

Time Estimate: 20 minutes active time, 1 hour inactive time

MAKES 6 JUMBO MUFFIN-SIZE BUNS

Do not double or halve

....

This recipe is an abbreviated version of the Cinnamon Buns recipe in my first book, *Gluten-Free on a Shoestring*. The buns are made in muffin cups, which helps support the dough, allowing for an easier rise and letting us rush the process a bit by adding more yeast. They still have that cinnamon goodness that we all love, and they're dairy-free! Feel free to sub back in dairy milk where the recipe calls for nondairy milk, though, if that's how you roll (get it?).

3 cups (420 g) high-quality all-purpose gluten-free flour

2¼ teaspoons xanthan gum (omit if your blend already contains it)

¼ teaspoon kosher salt, plus a dash (⅛ teaspoon) more for the filling

⅓ cup (67 g) granulated sugar

4 teaspoons instant yeast

¼ teaspoon cream of tartar

1½ teaspoons ground cinnamon

4 tablespoons (48 g) vegetable shortening

1 teaspoon pure vanilla extract

2 extra-large eggs, at room temperature, lightly beaten

1½ cups warm nondairy milk (about 100°F; I prefer unsweetened almond milk),
    plus 2 to 4 tablespoons more for the icing

2 tablespoons (28 g) grapeseed or canola oil

⅔ cup (145 g) light brown sugar

¾ cup (86 g) confectioners' sugar

1. Grease the wells of a jumbo six-cup muffin tin, and set the pan aside.

2. First, make the dough. Place the flour, xanthan gum, ¼ teaspoon of salt, the granulated sugar, yeast, and cream of tartar, and ½ teaspoon of the cinnamon in the bowl of your stand mixer fitted with the paddle attachment. Whisk well. Add the shortening, vanilla, and eggs, one at a time, mixing well after each addition.

3. With the mixer on low speed, add the 1½ cups of milk in a steady stream. The mixture should come together as dough. The dough should be very thick and smooth, and a bit tacky to the touch. If it seems wet, add more flour by the tablespoon until it is only tacky, but not wet. Turn out the dough onto a lightly floured surface and allow it to rest for a moment while you prepare the filling.

4. To make the filling, place the oil, light brown sugar, remaining teaspoon of cinnamon, and pinch of salt in a small bowl. Mix the ingredients well. The mixture will be grainy. Keep this mixture handy as you shape the dough.

5. To shape the dough, divide it into six equal pieces. With well-floured hands, shape each piece of dough into a cylinder about 6 inches long by rolling it back and forth on the lightly floured surface. Cover the dough with a piece of unbleached parchment paper, and roll each cylinder into a rectangle, 6 inches long and 1½ inches wide. As you work, if your hands stick to the dough, flour them. Repeat with the remaining pieces of dough. Line up the rectangles horizontally, like the stripes on the American flag, on a large piece of parchment paper.

6. Divide the filling evenly among the rectangles, gently pressing the filling into the dough so it doesn't come off as you roll the dough into buns. Next, roll each piece of dough as tightly as possible into a bun, from one short side of the rectangle to the other.

7. Place each bun into a well of the prepared muffin tin, and place the tin in a warm, moist, draft-free location to rise for about 30 minutes. Don't worry about its doubling in size. These are quicker buns.

8. As the buns are rising, preheat your oven to 350°F. Place the muffin tin in the center of the preheated oven and bake for about 30 minutes, or until the edges of the buns are lightly brown and the center is solid to the touch. If you bake them for too long, the bottoms of the buns will begin to burn. You have to judge the bottoms by what you see on the sides.

9. Allow the buns to cool completely before icing them, or the icing will melt and disappear right into the bun.

10. To make the icing as the buns are cooling, place the confectioners' sugar in a small bowl and add the remaining 2 tablespoons of milk, then mix well. The icing should be thick but pourable. Add more milk by the tablespoon and mix it in to reach the desired consistency. Once the buns are cool, pour or spread the icing on top of each bun. Serve immediately.

Quickest, Yeast-Free Cinnamon Buns

Time Estimate: 15 minutes active time, 25 minutes inactive time

MAKES 12 BUNS

Can be doubled or halved easily

....

Okay, now we're really talking quick. You really do need to make these in a standard twelve-cup muffin tin, or they will unravel and we will both be sad. I might not be there with you in person, but somehow, wherever you are, I will know. And I will mourn. Because it's happened to me. Learn from my mistakes.

3½ to 4 cups (490 to 560 g) high-quality all-purpose gluten-free flour

2 teaspoons xanthan gum (omit if your blend already contains it)

2½ teaspoons baking powder

⅜ teaspoon kosher salt

½ cup (100 g) granulated sugar

12 tablespoons (168 g) unsalted butter, at room temperature

2 extra-large eggs, at room temperature, lightly beaten

1 cup milk, at room temperature (low-fat is fine, nonfat is not)

1 cup (218 g) light brown sugar

2 tablespoons ground cinnamon

4 ounces mascarpone cheese, at room temperature

1½ cups (173 g) confectioners' sugar

1. Preheat your oven to 350°F. Grease the wells of a standard twelve-cup muffin tin and set it aside.

2. In a large bowl, place 3½ cups (490 g) of the flour, the xanthan gum, baking powder, ¼ teaspoon of the salt, and the granulated sugar, and whisk well. Add 6 tablespoons of the butter, the eggs, and the milk, and mix until the dough comes together. The dough should be smooth and relatively easy to handle. If the dough seems sticky, add more flour by the tablespoon and knead it in with well-floured hands until the dough is smooth.

3. Turn out the dough onto a piece of lightly floured unbleached parchment paper. Place another piece of parchment paper on top and roll the dough into a 10 by 15-inch rectangle, about ¼ inch thick (no thinner).

4. In a separate small bowl, place the brown sugar, cinnamon, 4 tablespoons of the butter, and the remaining ⅛ teaspoon of salt, and mix well. Set the bowl aside.

5. With a small offset spatula or large spoon, spread the cinnamon mixture in an even layer over the top of the dough, leaving about ¼ inch clean around the perimeter. Starting at a long side, roll the dough away from you into a tightly formed roll. Slice the roll in cross-section into twelve equal pieces, each about 1 inch thick. Place each roll in the well of the prepared muffin tin.

6. Place the tin in the center of the preheated oven, and bake for about 25 minutes, or until the rolls begin to turn golden brown and the filling starts to bubble out of them. Remove from the oven and allow to cool until the rolls are firm enough to handle, and transfer to a wire rack to finish cooling. Be sure to remove the rolls from the muffin tin before they are completely cool, or they will begin to stick to the baking pan.

7. While the rolls are cooling, make the icing. In a separate small bowl, mix together the mascarpone, the remaining 2 tablespoons of butter, and the confectioners' sugar until smooth but thickly pourable. Drizzle the icing on the rolls before serving.

Shoestring Savings

On a shoestring: 34¢ each

If you bought it: 67¢ each

No-Bake Berry Breakfast Protein Bars

Time Estimate: 10 minutes active time, 10 minutes inactive time
MAKES 16 SQUARE BARS
Can be doubled or halved easily

....

Between the nut butter and the protein powder, these pack quite the morning punch. Ever since I can remember, I've obsessed about my kids' having a source of high-quality protein in the mornings before school. That almost always means scrambled eggs with a splash of cream, but sometimes . . . I oversleep. It happens! I always have a supply of some sort of make-ahead protein bar in the refrigerator to toss at them, and you'll never hear them complaining. This one is a berry variety, but really you could use any sort of dried fruit you and your family like.

2½ cups (250 g) gluten-free old-fashioned rolled oats
1 cup (128 g) gluten-free whey powder (or any other type of gluten-free protein
     powder)
5 ounces (140 g) dried cranberries or blueberries (or a mixture of both)
¾ cup (200 g) no-stir smooth nut butter (such as Barney Butter Almond Butter or
     Peanut Butter & Co. Smooth Operator Peanut Butter)
2 tablespoons Lyle's golden syrup or honey
⅔ cup milk (low-fat is fine, nonfat is not)

1. Line a 9-inch square baking pan with unbleached parchment paper, large enough to overhang the sides of the dish, and set it aside.

2. If you'd like oats that are less chewy, place the oats in a blender or food processor, and grind or pulse until the oats are more processed by about half.

3. In a large bowl, place the oats, protein powder, and dried berries, and whisk well.

4. In a small saucepan, place the nut butter, syrup, and milk. Cook, stirring frequently, over medium-low heat until the nut butter and syrup are melted and the milk has begun to simmer, about 3 minutes. Pour the nut butter mixture over the dry ingredients, and mix well. The mixture will be very thick.

5. Use a wet spatula to scrape the mixture into the prepared baking dish and spread into an even layer. Freeze until firm, about 15 minutes.

6. Once firm, lift up the parchment paper to remove the contents from the pan, and place on a cutting board. Slice into sixteen squares with a sharp, wet knife. Store in an airtight container in the refrigerator until ready to use. They will last about a week in the refrigerator, and can also be frozen.

Shoestring Savings

On a shoestring: 50¢ each

If you bought it: $1.00 each

No-Bake Chocolate Breakfast Protein Bars

Time Estimate: 10 minutes active time, 10 minutes inactive time

MAKES 16 SQUARE BARS

Can be doubled or halved easily

....

I think of these bars as a make-ahead protein shake in kid-friendly hold-in-your-hand bar form. The chocolate chips could be replaced with chopped almonds or walnuts. This is one of those rare moments where I really do recommend Dutch-processed cocoa powder; it is not acidic like natural cocoa powder, so it simply tastes much better in a no-bake bar. That said, you can replace with an equal amount of natural cocoa powder and still get pretty good results.

2½ cups (250 g) gluten-free old-fashioned rolled oats

¾ cup (96 g) chocolate protein powder (any gluten-free chocolate variety, such as Tera's Whey Fair Trade Dark Chocolate)

6 tablespoons (30 g) Dutch-processed unsweetened cocoa powder

5 ounces (140 g) semisweet chocolate chips

¾ cup (200 g) no-stir smooth nut butter (such as Barney Butter Almond Butter or Peanut Butter & Co. Smooth Operator Peanut Butter)

2 tablespoons Lyle's golden syrup or honey

⅔ cup milk (low-fat is fine, nonfat is not)

1. Line a 9-inch square baking pan with unbleached parchment paper, large enough to overhang the sides of the dish, and set it aside.

2. If you'd like oats that are less chewy, place the oats in a blender or food processor, and grind or pulse until the oats are more processed by about half.

3. In a large bowl, place the oats, chocolate protein powder and cocoa powder, and whisk to combine well. Add the chocolate chips, and mix to combine.

4. In a small saucepan, place the nut butter, syrup, and milk, and cook, stirring frequently, over medium-low heat until the nut butter and syrup are melted and the milk has begun to simmer, about 3 minutes. Pour the nut butter mixture over the dry ingredients, and mix well. The mixture will be very thick.

5. Scrape into the prepared baking dish, and spread into an even layer with a wet spatula. Freeze until firm, about 10 minutes.

6. Once firm, lift up the parchment paper to remove the contents from the pan, and place on a cutting board. Slice into sixteen squares with a sharp, wet knife. Store in an airtight container in the refrigerator until ready to use. They will last about a week in the refrigerator. They can also be frozen.

Shoestring Savings

On a shoestring: 38¢ each

If you bought it: $2.50 each

Vegan Granola Protein Bites

Time Estimate: 10 minutes active time, 10 minutes inactive time

MAKES 20 BITES

Can be doubled or halved easily

....

I've grown quite fond of finely ground almond flour. It can be tricky to find a reliable vegan replacement for dairy whey protein powder, especially if you'd rather not use soy. Finely ground almond flour is a great alternative. You can grind your own, but for convenience I buy Barney Butter Almond Flour online. I like that it has a fine grain, is reliably gluten-free, and that it's a consistently good product. It's not cheap, though, so I use it sparingly.

2½ cups (250 g) gluten-free old-fashioned rolled oats

1 cup plus 2 tablespoons (126 g) finely ground almond flour

6 ounces (168 g) dried cranberries, blueberries, or golden raisins (or a blend)

¾ cup (200 g) no-stir smooth nut butter (such as Barney Butter Almond Butter or Peanut Butter & Co. Smooth Operator Peanut Butter)

2 tablespoons Lyle's golden syrup or honey

⅔ cup almond milk, or other nondairy milk

1. Preheat your oven to 375°F. Line a rimmed baking sheet with unbleached parchment paper and set it aside.

2. If you'd like oats that are less chewy, place the oats in a blender or food processor, and grind or pulse until the oats are more processed by about half.

3. Place the oats, almond flour, and dried berries in a large bowl and mix to combine well.

4. In a small saucepan, place the nut butter, syrup, and milk, and cook, stirring frequently, over medium-low heat until the nut butter and syrup are melted and the milk has begun to simmer, about 3 minutes. Pour the nut butter mixture over the dry ingredients, and mix well. The mixture will be very thick.

5. Divide the dough into twenty pieces, roll each into a ball and then flatten into a disk. Place about 1 inch apart on the prepared baking sheet. Bake the protein bites in the center of the oven until they are firm and just beginning to brown on the bottom, about 10 minutes.

6. Remove from the oven and allow to cool completely on the baking sheet. Store in an airtight container in the refrigerator until ready to use. They will last about 5 days in the refrigerator without drying out. They can also be frozen.

Shoestring Savings

On a shoestring: 30¢ each

If you bought it: $1.04 each

Pumpkin Granola Breakfast Cookies

Time Estimate: 10 minutes active time, 20 minutes inactive time

MAKES 36 BREAKFAST COOKIES

Can be doubled or halved easily

....

Cookies for breakfast? You'd better believe it. These soft pumpkin granola cookies are a snap to make, and easy to serve for breakfast because you make them ahead of time. I store them layered in an airtight container, with a piece of parchment paper between layers so they don't stick together. A little upfront work, a big morning rush payoff. If you don't have pumpkin pie spice on hand, you can make your own by whisking together 1 tablespoon of ground cinnamon, 1 teaspoon of ground nutmeg, 1 teaspoon of ground ginger, and ½ teaspoon of ground allspice.

2 cups (280 g) high-quality all-purpose gluten-free flour

1 teaspoon xanthan gum (omit if your blend already contains it)

1 teaspoon baking soda

1 teaspoon baking powder

½ teaspoon kosher salt

1 teaspoon ground cinnamon

1 teaspoon pumpkin pie spice

¼ cup (50 g) granulated sugar

½ cup (109 g) packed brown sugar

1¾ cups gluten-free granola (can be replaced by 1½ cups gluten-free
   old-fashioned rolled oats plus ¼ cup dried fruit)

1 tablespoon neutral oil (such as grapeseed or canola)

1 teaspoon pure vanilla extract

4 tablespoons (56 g) unsalted butter, at room temperature

2 extra-large eggs, at room temperature, lightly beaten

7½ ounces (half a 15-ounce can) pure packed pumpkin

1. Preheat your oven to 375°F. Line rimmed baking sheets with unbleached parchment paper and set them aside.

2. In a large bowl, place the flour, xanthan gum, baking soda, baking powder, salt, cinnamon, pumpkin pie spice, granulated sugar, and brown sugar, and whisk well, eliminating any lumps. Add the granola and mix again.

3. Add the oil, vanilla, butter, eggs, and pumpkin, mixing well after each addition. The batter will be thick and stiff, but not quite as stiff as you would expect regular cookie dough to be.

4. Divide the dough into thirty-six equal portions. This works best with a small, spring-loaded ice-cream scoop, but can easily be done with two small spoons. Place the portions of dough about 1 inch apart on the prepared baking sheets. Place the baking sheets in the freezer for about 10 minutes, until the dough is firm.

5. Bake the cookies in the center of the oven for 10 to 12 minutes, or until lightly browned around the edges and solid to the touch, rotating the baking sheet once during baking.

6. Allow to cool on the baking sheet for 5 minutes before transferring the cookies to wire racks to cool completely.

7. Store the cookies back to back, with small sheets of parchment paper between pairs of cookies, in airtight containers either on the counter or in the refrigerator. Refrigeration tends to dry out baked goods, but these cookies are moist enough that they can stand up to it well for about 5 days. They will last about 2 days at room temperature, and can also be frozen for about 2 months.

Chocolate Popovers

Time Estimate: 10 minutes active time, 30 minutes inactive time
MAKES 6 POPOVERS
Can be doubled or halved easily

....

Let's talk popover pans. You don't need a popover pan for 'em to pop. But that's not to say that the manner in which you bake them doesn't matter. You need deep wells (but not deep pockets—get it?). These little gems pop, even without yeast or a leavener such as baking powder or baking soda. That's because the hot oven air circulates around the batter in the wells. Not much air circulation going on around shallow wells. So you can use a muffin tin with deep wells, or you can use individual baking cups. Those work, too. So glad we had this talk.

¾ cup (105 g) high-quality all-purpose gluten-free flour

Scant ½ teaspoon xanthan gum (omit if your blend already contains it)

½ teaspoon kosher salt

3 tablespoons (15 g) unsweetened natural cocoa powder

⅛ teaspoon baking soda

5 tablespoons (63 g) sugar

1 tablespoon (14 g) unsalted butter, melted and cooled

2 extra-large eggs, at room temperature, lightly beaten

1 cup milk, at room temperature (low-fat is fine, nonfat is not)

1. Preheat your oven to 375°F. Grease a six-cup popover pan (or six to eight cups, depending upon the size of the wells, of a muffin tin with deep wells) and set it aside.

2. In a large bowl, place the flour, xanthan gum, salt, cocoa powder, baking soda, and sugar, and whisk well. Add the butter, eggs, and milk, and mix well until smooth.

3. Divide the mixture among the prepared muffin cups and place the tin in the center of the preheated oven. Bake for about 30 minutes, or until puffed and firm to the touch on top.

4. After the first 20 minutes, quickly open the oven, and with a sharp knife or with sharp kitchen shears, pierce the top of each popover to allow steam to escape and the popovers to maintain their puffiness.

Shoestring Savings

On a shoestring: 25¢ each

If you bought it: 69¢ each

Egg in the Hole

Time Estimate: 15 minutes
MAKES 4 SERVINGS
Can be doubled or halved easily

....

This is so easy that it's barely a "recipe," so think of it more as an idea generator. The idea is that you can take something simple, such as a thick slice of bread, and dress it up into a nice breakfast. One of my children doesn't like the yolk this way, so I just remove it. Do you think I'm spoiling her by catering to her like that? Don't answer. Okay, tell me. No, don't answer.

4 thick (¾-inch) slices gluten-free bread (such as Quick-Rising Cornmeal
     Sandwich Bread, page 66)
4 extra-large eggs
About 4 tablespoons (48 g) unsalted butter
Kosher salt and freshly ground black pepper

1. With a 2-inch round biscuit or cookie cutter, cut a hole in the dead center of each slice of bread, and set the bread slices and cutouts aside.

2. Crack each of the eggs carefully into its own small bowl, and set the bowls aside.

3. Place about a tablespoon of butter in a 12-inch nonstick skillet. Melt the butter over medium heat and turn the pan to coat it with the melted butter. Place two slices of the bread, plus the round cutouts, in the skillet. Slide an egg into each hole. If you prefer well-cooked yolks, scoop out the yolks first and place them (whole) in the skillet as well. Salt and pepper the eggs to taste. Cook each slice for about a minute, until the egg whites have begun to set.

4. With a wide spatula, flip over the bread with the egg inside, and cook for about another minute, or until the bread is browned all over and the egg is set. If you have left the yolk with the white, it will be slightly runny. If you separated out the yolk, turn it over to cook fully. Be sure to flip the round cutouts of bread until they are browned on both sides.

5. Repeat the process with the other two slices of bread and two eggs. Serve immediately.

German Pancake

Time Estimate: 10 minutes active time, 20 minutes inactive time
MAKES 4 SERVINGS
Can be doubled or halved easily

....

Whether you call it a German Pancake or a Dutch Baby, this little darlin' is like a cross between the perfect popover and a lovely blintz pancake. It's crusty on the outside, soft and pillowy on the inside, and it all cooks up in minutes. The ingredients really do need to be at room temperature, but that doesn't mean this can't be a weekday breakfast for the whole family. Simply leave the eggs and milk out on the counter right before going to bed, and then wake up and just combine everything and pop it in the oven. While you get yourself ready for the day, breakfast is coming to life in a hot oven. If you have a choice between underbaking and overbaking the pancake, overbake it. Underbaked, it will deflate. Overbaked by a bit, it will just be a little crustier.

2 tablespoons (24 g) vegetable shortening
6 extra-large eggs, at room temperature, lightly beaten
1¼ cups milk at room temperature (low-fat is fine, nonfat is not)
1 cup (140 g) high-quality all-purpose gluten-free flour
¼ teaspoon xanthan gum (omit if your blend already contains it)
¼ teaspoon kosher salt
Confectioners' sugar, for dusting

1. Preheat your oven to 375°F. As the oven is heating, place the vegetable shortening in a 13 by 9 by 2-inch baking dish, and place the dish in the oven until the shortening melts (a few minutes, tops). Remove the baking dish from the oven, rotate it to distribute the shortening evenly around the pan, and set it aside.

2. In a large bowl, place the eggs, milk, flour, xanthan gum, and salt, and beat with a wire whisk until smooth and thickened. The batter will still be thin and pourable, but it should not be watery.

3. Pour the batter into the prepared baking dish and return it to the preheated oven. Bake for 18 to 20 minutes, rotating after 10 minutes, until the pancake is very puffy and the edges are golden brown.

4. Dust lightly with confectioners' sugar, slice into wedges, and enjoy right away.

Chocolate Breakfast Muffins

Time Estimate: 10 minutes active time, 25 minutes inactive time

MAKES 12 MUFFINS

Can be doubled or halved easily

....

These lightly sweet muffins have a subtle enough cocoa taste that you won't think you've gone and mistaken dessert for breakfast (or breakfast for dessert, for that matter). If you are so inclined, as I am, add some peppermint extract in place of the vanilla extract, and enjoy a muffin along with a piping hot cup of freshly brewed coffee.

1½ cups (210 g) high-quality all-purpose gluten-free flour

¾ teaspoon xanthan gum (omit if your blend already contains it)

⅔ cup (53 g) unsweetened natural cocoa powder

¼ teaspoon ground cinnamon

1½ teaspoons baking powder

½ teaspoon baking soda

½ teaspoon kosher salt

¾ cup (164 g) packed light brown sugar

8 tablespoons (112 g) unsalted butter, at room temperature

2 extra-large eggs, at room temperature, lightly beaten

1 cup plus 2 tablespoons buttermilk, at room temperature (low-fat is fine, nonfat
    is not)

1½ teaspoons pure vanilla extract (or replace with peppermint extract for choco-
    late mint muffins)

1. Preheat your oven to 350°F. Grease or line a standard twelve-cup muffin pan and set it aside.

2. In a large bowl, place the flour, xanthan gum, cocoa powder, cinnamon, baking powder, baking soda, salt, and brown sugar, and whisk well, working out any lumps in the brown sugar. Add the butter, eggs, buttermilk, and vanilla, stirring well after each addition.

3. Fill the muffin cups about three-quarters of the way full with batter. Bake the muffins for 20 to 25 minutes, rotating the tin once during baking. When done, a toothpick inserted into the center of a middle muffin should come out clean.

4. Allow to cool for at least 10 minutes before serving.

Shoestring Savings

On a shoestring: 34¢ each

If you bought it: $1.97 each

Yeast-Free Glazed Plain Doughnuts

Time Estimate: 20 minutes active time, 9 minutes inactive time
MAKES 15 MINI DOUGHNUTS
Can be doubled or halved easily

....

More often than not, I make these and the Yeast-Free Glazed Chocolate Dough-nuts (page 44) in that most ridiculous of contraptions that somehow found its way into my kitchen, the Babycakes Mini Doughnut Maker. Normally I'm not a fan of kitchen appliances that serve only one purpose, but that little machine heats up in no time. And even though I have to run its four-minute cycle at least three times to make a whole recipe, at least I'm eating a perfect, warm doughnut in about fifteen minutes flat, from conception to reality. How's that for quick and easy?

If you don't have a mini doughnut maker, though, fear not. You can make these in the oven as described in the recipe for Yeast-Free Glazed Chocolate Doughnuts (page 44)!

1¾ cups (245 g) high-quality all-purpose gluten-free flour

¾ teaspoon xanthan gum (omit if your blend already contains it)

1½ teaspoons baking powder

¼ teaspoon baking soda

¼ teaspoon cream of tartar

¼ teaspoon kosher salt

½ teaspoon freshly grated nutmeg

¾ cup (150 g) granulated sugar

4 tablespoons (56 g) unsalted butter, melted and cooled

4 tablespoons (48 g) vegetable shortening, melted and cooled

2 extra-large eggs, at room temperature, lightly beaten

1½ teaspoons pure vanilla extract

¾ cup plain yogurt, at room temperature

1 cup (115 g) confectioners' sugar

2 to 4 teaspoons milk or buttermilk

1. Warm the doughnut maker according to the manufacturer's directions.

2. In a large bowl, place the flour, xanthan gum, baking powder, baking soda, cream of tartar, salt, nutmeg, and sugar, and whisk well. Add the butter, shortening, eggs, vanilla, and yogurt, mixing to combine after each addition.

3. Fill the bottom of the doughnut wells completely with batter, then close and secure the lid. Allow to bake for 3 minutes. Open the doughnut maker and remove the doughnuts with the remover tool included in the package. Transfer to a wire rack to cool completely, and repeat with the remaining doughnut batter.

4. While the doughnuts are cooling, make the glaze. Have ready a piece of unbleached parchment paper. In a small bowl, place the confectioners' sugar and 2 teaspoons of the milk and mix well. Add more milk by the half-teaspoon until you have a smooth but thickly pourable liquid. Working quickly, dip the top of each slightly cooled doughnut in the glaze, turn back and forth a bit to coat well, invert so the glaze is facing upward, and allow to set on the parchment paper.

5. The glaze seals in moisture, so the glazed doughnuts will keep quite well uncovered on the counter for a few days. Freeze any unglazed leftovers.

Shoestring Savings

On a shoestring: 27¢ each

If you bought it: 80¢ each

Yeast-Free Glazed Chocolate Doughnuts

Time Estimate: 20 minutes active time, 8 minutes inactive time

MAKES 15 MINI DOUGHNUTS

Can be doubled or halved easily

If we've met before online, you and I have already talked about these chocolate doughnuts. When you bite into your first one, you'll see that it was worth the wait. These are moist but firm, and taste just as you want them to taste—chocolaty, but not like brownies. The hint of nutmeg in these and the Yeast-Free Glazed Plain Doughnuts (page 42) is owed to Lara Ferroni of *Doughnuts: Simple and Delicious Recipes to Make at Home.* She rightly says that it's what gives dough-nuts their, well, doughnut-ness (it is, too, a word!).

1½ cups (210 g) high-quality all-purpose gluten-free flour

¾ teaspoon xanthan gum (omit if your blend already contains it)

7 tablespoons (35 g) unsweetened natural cocoa powder

1½ teaspoons baking powder

¼ teaspoon baking soda

¼ teaspoon cream of tartar

¼ teaspoon kosher salt

½ teaspoon freshly grated nutmeg

⅔ cup (145 g) packed light brown sugar

4 tablespoons (56 g) unsalted butter, melted and cooled

4 tablespoons (55 g) canola oil

2 extra-large eggs, at room temperature, lightly beaten

1½ teaspoons pure vanilla extract

¾ cup plus 2 tablespoons (14 tablespoons) heavy cream, at room temperature

1 cup (115 g) confectioners' sugar

2 to 4 teaspoons milk or buttermilk

    1. Preheat your oven to 350°F. Grease a mini doughnut pan or muffin tin and set it aside.

    2. In a large bowl, place the flour, xanthan gum, 6 tablespoons of the cocoa powder, and the baking powder, baking soda, cream of tartar, salt, nutmeg, and

brown sugar, and whisk well. Add the butter, oil, eggs, vanilla, and cream, mixing to combine after each addition.

3. Fill the prepared doughnut or muffin wells about three-quarters of the way full. Place in the center of the oven and bake for about 10 minutes, or until the doughnuts are set and just lightly browned. Transfer to a wire rack to cool.

4. While the doughnuts are baking (or cooling), make the glaze. In a small bowl, place the confectioners' sugar, remaining 1 tablespoon of cocoa powder, and 2 teaspoons of milk, and mix well. Add more milk by the half-teaspoon until you have a smooth but thickly pourable liquid. Working quickly, dip the top of each slightly cooled doughnut in the glaze, turn back and forth a bit to coat well, invert so the glaze is facing upward, and allow it to set on a piece of parchment paper.

5. The glaze seals in moisture, so the glazed doughnuts will keep quite well uncovered on the counter for a few days. Freeze any unglazed leftovers.

VARIATION: Bake these doughnuts in a BabyCakes Mini Doughnut Maker. Instead of preheating your oven, warm the doughnut maker according to the manufacturer's directions. Follow Step 2 above to make the batter. In Step 3, fill the bottom of the doughnut maker wells completely with batter, then close and secure the lid. Allow to bake for 3 minutes. Open the doughnut maker and remove the doughnuts with the remover tool included in the package. Transfer to a wire rack to cool completely, and return to Step 4 of the recipe.

Shoestring Savings

On a shoestring: 33¢ each
If you bought it: 80¢ each

Breakfast Burritos

Time Estimate: 30 minutes (less if you use prepared corn tortillas)

MAKES 4 TO 6 SERVINGS

Can be doubled or halved easily

....

I cannot get enough of breakfast burritos, huevos rancheros, and Tex-Mex breakfasts built around the humble egg. Maybe I wish I were a rancher or something. (But I'm not using an outhouse, and I need clean sheets. I should probably just stick to making the food.)

4 extra-large eggs, lightly beaten

1 tablespoon heavy cream

1 medium-size onion, peeled and diced

2 tablespoons extra-virgin olive oil

1 teaspoon ground cumin

½ teaspoon Mexican chili powder, or to taste

Kosher salt

Freshly ground black pepper

1 recipe Flour Tortillas (page 80), kept warm, or 8 corn tortillas, moistened and
     warmed in the microwave oven until pliable

6 to 8 ounces Monterey Jack cheese, grated

2 medium-size tomatoes, seeded and chopped

1 ripe avocado, pitted and diced (optional)

Prepared salsa, for serving

1. In a small bowl, place the eggs and cream, and beat well. In a large nonstick skillet over medium heat, cook the eggs, stirring frequently, until slightly runny. Remove from the skillet and set aside.

2. In the same skillet, sauté the onions in the olive oil over medium-high heat, stirring frequently, until the onions are translucent, about 6 minutes. Add the cumin, chili powder, and salt and pepper, and stir well. Remove the pan from the heat.

3. Open the first tortilla, sprinkle with a bit of cheese, and place about one-sixth of the eggs across the center of the tortilla. Top with some chopped tomatoes

and more grated cheese. Fold in the sides of the tortilla, and roll away from you until the tortilla is sealed. Press down lightly.

4. Repeat with the remaining tortillas. Microwave each tortilla on HIGH for about 45 seconds, or until the cheese is fully melted and has sealed the burrito closed.

5. Allow to set briefly before serving, scattered with the chopped avocado (if using) and salsa on the side.

Shoestring Savings

On a shoestring: $1.03 each

If you bought it: $3.44 each (frozen)

Texas Toast

Time Estimate: 10 minutes active time
MAKES 4 SERVINGS
Can be doubled or halved easily

....

I think you're meant to make Texas Toast with monster-size slices of packaged bread. Last I checked, there is no such thing in Gluten-Free-Land. No mind. We can make our own bread, thank you very much. But if someone does come out with a packaged gluten-free bread that's just right for Texas Toast, believe me when I say I'll be first in line to give it a try.

About 6 tablespoons (84 g) unsalted butter
4 thick (¾-inch) slices gluten-free bread (such as Quick-Rising
    Cornmeal Sandwich Bread, page 66)

1. Line a rimmed baking sheet with unbleached parchment paper and set it aside.

2. In a 12-inch cast-iron or nonstick skillet, place 3 tablespoons of butter. Melt the butter over medium heat, and turn the pan to coat it with the melted butter. Place two slices of bread in the skillet, and cook until the bread starts to brown. With a wide spatula, flip the bread over, and cook for about another minute, or until the bread is browned all over. Slice the bread in half diagonally to create tri-angles. Place the slices in a single layer on the prepared baking sheet.

3. Repeat with the remaining two slices of bread, and the remaining butter.

4. Turn on your oven's broiler, and place the baking sheet about 3 inches from the flame. Broil until golden brown on one side, about 2 minutes, flip the slices over, and repeat the process on the other side. Serve immediately.

Muesli

Time Estimate: 25 minutes
MAKES 6 ½ CUPS, OR 4 TO 6 SERVINGS
Can be doubled or halved easily

Rice bran adds fiber and some heft to this Swiss cousin of oatmeal. Some like to soak a serving of muesli in milk overnight in the refrigerator before eating. I'm one of those some. And you'll find plenty of other uses for that rice bran, some are on my blog in my ready-to-eat cereal recipes and bran muffins.

3½ cups (350 g) gluten-free old-fashioned rolled oats
½ cup (65 g) raw pecans
½ cup (72 g) raw whole almonds
½ cup (30 g) unsweetened coconut chips
½ cup (120 g) dried apricots
½ cup (92 g) dried blueberries or golden raisins
¾ cup (90 g) gluten-free stabilized rice bran

1. Preheat your oven to 325°F. Line a rimmed baking sheet with unbleached parchment paper and place the oats on it in an even layer. Bake, stirring occasionally to prevent burning, until golden brown, about 12 minutes. Transfer the oats to a large, heat-safe bowl.

2. Place the pecans and almonds on the same prepared baking sheet in an even layer and bake until very lightly toasted, about 5 minutes. Add the nuts to the bowl of oats. Toss well.

3. Place the coconut chips on the baking sheet in an even layer and bake until some of the chips are golden brown and toasted, about 5 minutes. Add the coconut to the bowl of nuts and oats. Toss well.

4. Add the dried fruit and the rice bran to the bowl of nuts, oats, and coconut chips, and toss again. Store in an airtight container until ready to use. Serve with yogurt or milk, and drizzle with honey if desired.

Shoestring Savings

On a shoestring: 50¢ per serving

If you bought it: $1.00 per serving

Morning Polenta

Time Estimate: 10 minutes

MAKES 4 SERVINGS

Can be doubled or halved easily

....

De la Estancia brand organic polenta is not marketed as quick-cooking. But it's finely ground and cooks in about a minute. It's a polenta miracle! And it's from Italy. Somehow, I find that comforting. For this recipe, consider everything to be suggestions, except of course, for what you need to make the actual polenta. This polenta will stand up to whatever sweet or savory add-ins are your favorite. The versatility alone makes it a sure-fire crowd-pleaser.

1½ cups milk (low-fat is fine, nonfat is not)

1½ cups water

1 cup (170 g) De la Estancia organic polenta

¼ teaspoon kosher salt

¼ cup (55 g) packed light brown sugar, plus more for serving

½ teaspoon pure vanilla extract

Dried fruit, for serving

Ground cinnamon, for dusting

1. Place the milk and water in a medium-size stockpot. Bring to a boil over medium-high heat. Turn down the heat to medium-low and gradually stir in the polenta and the salt.

2. Cook, stirring constantly, for 1 minute, or until thickened and beginning to pull away from the sides of the stockpot. Add the ¼ cup of brown sugar and the vanilla, and stir well.

3. Divide the polenta among four bowls, sprinkle each with more brown sugar, and serve immediately with dried fruit and a dusting of cinnamon.

Baked Oatmeal

Time Estimate: 5 minutes active time, 35 minutes inactive time
MAKES 4 SERVINGS
Can be doubled or halved easily

....

I would like to say a personal thank-you to the companies that grow and process oats in a dedicated gluten-free environment. I remember being giddy with excitement when I first learned years ago that anyone was doing that. I hurried up and made my family some good old-fashioned celiac-safe oatmeal. My son, the backward celiac who rejects rice nearly outright, added oatmeal to his list of dislikes. Thankfully, he's since righted this grievous wrong, and happily eats oatmeal. I think this baked version would help to win over even the pickiest toddler. You'd have to let me know, though, as I have no toddlers left to experiment upon.

1½ cups (150 g) gluten-free old-fashioned rolled oats

¼ teaspoon baking soda

¾ cup (138 g) dried blueberries or cherries

2 tablespoons (28 g) canola oil

¼ cup pure maple syrup (preferably Grade B)

2 cups milk (low-fat is fine, nonfat is not)

1. Preheat your oven to 375°F. Grease a 9-inch square pan and set it aside.

2. If you'd like oats that are less chewy, place the oats in a blender or food processor, and grind or pulse until the oats are more processed by about half.

3. Place the oats and baking soda in a large bowl, and mix well. Add the dried fruit and toss to coat.

4. In a separate small bowl, whisk together the oil, maple syrup, and milk. Create a well in the center of the oat mixture and pour in the milk mixture. Mix until just incorporated.

5. Scrape the oatmeal into the prepared pan and spread into an even layer with a wet spoon or spatula.

6. Bake the oatmeal in the center of the oven until the liquid has been absorbed and the edges are beginning to brown, about 35 minutes. Serve warm.

VARIATION: For Chocolate Baked Oatmeal, add ¼ cup (20 g) of unsweetened natural cocoa powder before adding the baking soda, and proceed with the recipe as written.

Drop Biscuits

Time Estimate: 10 minutes active time, 15 minutes inactive time
MAKES 8 BISCUITS
Can be doubled or halved easily

....

If you want a biscuit filled with layer after flaky layer, you are going to have to roll out the dough and treat it almost like you would the Quick Puff Pastry (page 82). But if all you're after is a light and tender biscuit, a drop biscuit should do you just fine. Just make this supereasy dough, drop it in mounds on a baking sheet and give it a quick spin in the oven. Once again, how's that for quick and easy?

2 cups (280 g) high-quality all-purpose gluten-free flour
1 teaspoon xanthan gum (omit if your blend already contains it)
1 tablespoon baking powder
¼ teaspoon baking soda
2 teaspoons sugar
½ teaspoon kosher salt
8 tablespoons (112 g) unsalted butter, roughly chopped and chilled
1 cup milk (low-fat is fine, nonfat is not), chilled
1½ teaspoons white wine vinegar

1. Preheat your oven to 400°F. Line a rimmed baking sheet with unbleached parchment paper and set it aside.

2. In a large bowl, place the flour, xanthan gum, baking powder, baking soda, sugar, and salt, and whisk well.

3. Add the cold, chopped butter, and toss to coat it with the dry ingredients. With well-floured fingers, press each piece of butter firmly between your thumb and forefinger to flatten.

4. Create a well in the center of the mixture and pour in the milk and vinegar. Stir to incorporate. The mixture should come together but still be wet. Using a 1½-inch spring-loaded ice-cream scoop, scoop out eight mounds of dough and drop each onto the prepared baking sheet, about 1 inch apart from one another.

5. Place the biscuits in the center of the preheated oven and bake, rotating once, until pale golden, about 15 minutes. Remove from the oven and allow to cool on the baking sheet before serving.

Chapter 4

Breads: Quicker and Quickest

YEAST-FREE SANDWICH BREADS AND
RAPID-RISE YEAST BREADS

We have bread now. We do! We can buy gluten-free bread at health food stores and in large chains, such as Whole Foods. And it's not half bad. It looks like bread and tastes like bread. Hurray!

But you know and I know that there's still some pretty serious deprivation going on. I don't mean to complain, except much of the gluten-free bread that's out there is small in size and priced high. It's not a complete answer. And there are still plenty of holes in the market, such as for ready-made wonton skins and more varieties of soft and pliable gluten-free flour tortillas. So don't put away your pizza stone just yet. We still need to bake bread.

No one loves yeast bread more than I do, but it's not always practical. And I've found that I've been able to make yeast-free versions of gluten-free English muffins (page 55) and gluten-free pita bread (page 57) that are so good, not only won't you miss the yeast, but you may even come to rely upon them as a cornerstone of your weekday dinners. And nothing beats yeasted refrigerator bread dough for a fresh yet impromptu dinner roll.

- ⚜ Yeast-Free English Muffins
- ⚜ Yeast-Free Pita Bread
- ⚜ Yeast-Free Hamburger Buns

- Yeast-Free Sandwich Bread
- Yeasted Refrigerator Pizza Dough
- Yeast-Free Pizza Dough
- Quick-Rising Cornmeal Sandwich Bread
- Quick-Rising Oatmeal Molasses Bread
- Yeasted Refrigerator Bread Dough
- Boule Bread with Yeasted Refrigerator Bread Dough
- Dinner Rolls with Yeasted Refrigerator Bread Dough
- Saltine-Style Crackers
- Goldfish-Style Crackers
- Pan de Bono
- Flour Tortillas
- Quick Puff Pastry
- Garlic Parmesan Breadsticks
- Basic Pastry Crust

Yeast-Free English Muffins

Time Estimate: 15 minutes active time, 15 minutes inactive time

MAKES 6 FULL-SIZE MUFFINS

Can be doubled or halved

You know how beautiful these are. You can see for yourself in the photos. But what you maybe can't see is how authentic they taste—or how speedy they are to make. Freeze a batch and you'll have them on hand all week for breakfast. Be sure to pick up a few English muffin rings. I have a couple of sets made by Fox Run, and they come in very handy since they force the muffins to rise up instead of out.

2 cups (280 g) high-quality all-purpose gluten-free flour

1 teaspoon xanthan gum (omit if your blend already contains it)

¼ teaspoon baking soda

1¼ teaspoons baking powder

2 teaspoons (8 g) sugar

1 teaspoon kosher salt

2 tablespoons (24 g) vegetable shortening, melted and cooled

1 teaspoon apple cider vinegar

1 extra-large egg, at room temperature, lightly beaten

1 cup milk, at room temperature (low-fat is fine, nonfat is not)

1. Preheat your oven to 400°F. Grease the inside of six English muffin rings and set them aside. Line a rimmed baking sheet with unbleached parchment paper and set it aside.

2. In a large bowl, place the flour, xanthan gum, baking soda, baking powder, sugar, and salt, and whisk well.

3. Add the 2 tablespoons of melted shortening, vinegar, egg, and milk, mixing to combine after each addition. The dough should come together and be soft and a bit slick.

4. With wet hands and a bench scraper, divide the dough into six equal portions. Wet your hands once more, and gently press each portion into a disk about the size and shape of one of the muffin rings.

5. Heat a cast-iron or other heavy-bottomed skillet on the stovetop over high heat. Place as many greased rings in the skillet as will fit comfortably. Drop a disk of dough in the center of each ring. Sear for a few moments on the first side, or until it begins to develop some color on the underside. Then flip each muffin with a wide spatula and sear the other side. Transfer the seared muffins (in their rings) to the prepared baking sheet and set aside. Repeat with the remaining muffins, if any.

6. Place the baking sheet with the English muffins in the center of the preheated oven and bake for 15 minutes. Remove the rings and bake the muffins for another 5 minutes, or until the muffins are lightly browned on the sides. Serve the same day, or split them and freeze for later use.

Shoestring Savings

On a shoestring: 44¢ each

If you bought it: $1.57 each

Yeast-Free Pita Bread

Time Estimate: 15 minutes active time, 15 minutes inactive time
MAKES 6 PITAS
Can be doubled or halved easily

··

These puff, but they don't "pop" like their yeasted cousins. No mind. Slice one open on a cutting board and then do surgery to create a pocket. Like the Yeast-Free English Muffins (page 55), they, too, are weeknight-dinner-friendly. My family and I love them with Baked Falafel (page 104), but they're right at home stuffed with a quick Greek salad, too.

2 cups (280 g) high-quality all-purpose gluten-free flour

1 teaspoon xanthan gum (omit if your blend already contains it)

1½ teaspoons baking powder

1 teaspoon kosher salt

1 tablespoon vegetable oil

1 extra-large egg plus 1 extra-large egg white, at room temperature, lightly
    beaten

¼ cup milk, at room temperature (low-fat is fine, nonfat is not)

½ to ¾ cup water, at room temperature

1. Preheat your oven to 400°F. If you have a pizza stone, place it in the oven while the oven heats up. If not, use an overturned rimmed baking sheet.

2. In the bowl of your stand mixer fitted with the paddle attachment or the bowl of your food processor, place the flour, xanthan gum, baking powder, and salt. Mix (or pulse) well.

3. Add the oil, eggs, and milk. Mix (or pulse) to incorporate. Then, with the mixer on its lowest speed (or the food processor on), add ½ cup of the water in a slow and steady stream. The dough will be wet. Mix until the dough is fluffy. Only parts of the dough will begin to pull away from the sides of the bowl, but it will not clump. If it doesn't seem quite wet enough, add water by the tablespoon.

4. Scrape the dough out of the bowl and place it on a wet, smooth surface (such as a wet Silpat or wet pastry board—a wet, smooth countertop will do, too). Divide

the dough into six equal parts (each about 90 grams) with a wet bench scraper. With wet hands (I know; stop saying wet, Nicole), form one piece of dough into a ball. Place the dough on a sheet of unbleached parchment paper, and with very wet fingertips, smooth the dough in a circular motion, adding some pressure to form it into a round, about ½ inch thick. Repeat with the remaining pieces of dough, placed about ½ inch apart on the parchment paper.

5. Place the dough, already on the parchment paper, in the oven atop the hot pizza stone (or overturned rimmed baking sheet). Bake for 5 minutes. Carefully flip the pitas and bake for another 5 to 7 minutes, or until lightly browned on both sides.

6. Remove the pitas from the oven and allow to cool for 3 to 5 minutes, or until they can be handled. Slice each round in half through the center. With a very sharp knife, gently coax open the center of each pita half.

7. Serve warm or at room temperature. Once cooled, the pitas will keep for 2 days in a resealable plastic bag at room temperature.

Shoestring Savings

On a shoestring: 42¢ each, or $2.49 for 6

If you bought it: $1.50 each, or $9 for 6

Yeast-Free Hamburger Buns

Time Estimate: 15 minutes active time, 45 minutes inactive time
MAKES 10 TO 12 BUNS
Can be doubled or halved somewhat easily

....

Having a burger without the bun is not really like having a burger. These buns are
so quick and easy to make, you won't have to pretend to be satisfied with just a
burger, hold the bun. They will rise, and then fall a bit as they cool. If you want
them to hold their shape a bit better, just bake them a little longer. They may
blacken a bit around the edges, but they won't taste burned. It's just the sugar,
toasting. And finally, although I call these Hamburger Buns, they're here for all
your bun-type needs.

2½ cups (350 g) high-quality all-purpose gluten-free flour

1¾ teaspoons xanthan gum (omit if your blend already contains it)

½ cup (58 g) confectioners' sugar

1½ teaspoons baking powder

½ teaspoon baking soda

Scant ½ cup (43 g) cultured buttermilk blend powder (I use Saco brand), or ⅓
    cup (43 g) whey powder

¼ teaspoon cream of tartar

½ teaspoon kosher salt

Finely grated zest of 1 medium-size lemon (optional)

¾ teaspoon apple cider vinegar

5 extra-large eggs, at room temperature, lightly beaten

½ cup milk, at room temperature (low-fat is fine, nonfat is not)

12 tablespoons (168 g) unsalted butter, melted and cooled

1. Preheat your oven to 375°F. Line rimmed baking sheets with unbleached
parchment paper and set them aside.

2. In the bowl of a stand mixer fitted with the paddle attachment, place the
flour, xanthan gum, sugar, baking powder, baking soda, buttermilk powder, cream

of tartar, and salt. Whisk with a separate handheld whisk until well combined. Add the lemon zest (if using) and whisk to incorporate into the dry ingredients.

3. Add the cider vinegar, eggs, milk, and butter, mixing well on low speed after each addition. Once the butter has been mixed in, beat at high speed for about 5 minutes, or until the mixture is pale yellow and thickened. The batter will be smooth and thick, but not stiff.

4. Divide the dough with a spoon into ten to twelve parts. With very, very wet hands, shape each portion of dough into a round and then flatten until ¾ inch to 1 inch thick. Place on the prepared baking sheets, arranging about 2 inches apart.

5. Place in the center of the preheated oven and bake for 15 minutes. Lower the temperature to 325°F and bake for another 25 to 35 minutes or more, depending upon how browned you would like the outside. Rotate the baking sheet once during baking, and when rotating, with a sharp knife or kitchen shears, cut a small slit in the top of each bun to allow some steam to escape. This will help keep the buns from deflating too much upon cooling.

6. Allow the buns to cool for at least 10 minutes before slicing them in the center and serving. They will deflate a bit after baking.

Shoestring Savings

On a shoestring: 50¢ each, or $2.00 for 4

If you bought it: $1.75 each, or $7.00 for 4

Yeast-Free Sandwich Bread

Time Estimate: 15 minutes active time, 50 minutes inactive time
MAKES 1 LOAF OF BREAD
Should not be doubled or halved, but can be frozen

Who says sandwich breads can't be quick breads? I thought there must have been some top-secret expert commando reason why I never, ever saw sandwich breads made yeast-free, much less gluten-free. Guess what? They can! Instead of waiting at least 40 minutes for yeast bread to rise before you can bake it, you can have this bread on your table in about an hour, start to finish.

4 extra-large egg whites, at room temperature

¼ teaspoon cream of tartar

3 cups (420 g) high-quality all-purpose gluten-free flour

1½ teaspoons xanthan gum (omit if your blend already contains it)

1 teaspoon kosher salt

5 tablespoons (40 g) whey powder

4 teaspoons baking powder

6 tablespoons (84 g) unsalted butter, at room temperature

2 tablespoons honey

2 teaspoons apple cider vinegar

1½ cups milk, at room temperature (low-fat is fine, nonfat is not)

1. Preheat your oven to 375°F. Grease well a 9 by 5-inch loaf pan and set it aside.

2. In the bowl of your stand mixer fitted with the whisk attachment, beat two of the egg whites on high speed until stiff (but not dry) peaks form, adding the cream of tartar about halfway through. Using a silicone spatula, gently scrape the beaten egg whites into a medium-size bowl and set aside.

3. Fit the stand mixer with the paddle attachment. Again in the bowl of your mixer, place the flour, xanthan gum, salt, whey powder, and baking powder. One at a time, add the butter, honey, vinegar, two remaining egg whites, and milk to the dry ingredients, mixing well after each addition.

4. Beat on low speed until the dry and wet ingredients begin to come together. Raise the speed, and beat until the mixture becomes smooth. It will be stiff and thick. Add one-third of the egg whites to the dough and mix slowly, using the paddle attachment, until the egg whites are just incorporated into the batter.

5. Remove the bowl from the mixer and gently fold the remaining egg whites into the batter by hand until nearly no white streaks remain. It is more important that the egg whites not get deflated than it is to rid the batter of every white streak. If a few white streaks remain, so be it.

6. With a spatula, scrape the dough into the prepared loaf pan. Wet the spatula and use it to smooth out the top of the batter gently. Grease the underside of a piece of aluminum foil with cooking spray, and tent the loaf pan with the foil.

7. Place the loaf pan in the center of the preheated oven and bake for about 45 minutes, rotating once during baking. Remove the foil and continue to bake until the top is browned and a toothpick inserted into the center comes out clean, about another 5 minutes. Allow the bread to cool for a few minutes in the pan, and then turn out onto a wire rack to cool completely before slicing.

Shoestring Savings

On a shoestring: $2.16 for a 12-ounce loaf

If you bought it: $7.08 for a 12-ounce loaf

Yeasted Refrigerator Pizza Dough

Time Estimate: 10 minutes active time, 40 minutes inactive time
MAKES ENOUGH CRUST FOR TWO 12-INCH PIZZAS
Can be halved (but not doubled) easily

···

This is a variation on the Pizza Dough recipe from *Gluten-Free on a Shoestring*. But this time around, I'm here to tell you that you can (and, I submit, should) make some on Sunday, and have it in the refrigerator for most of the week. It will rise very slowly in the refrigerator, leading to a more complex yeast flavor. Once you have a refrigerator stock of this on hand, you're never more than about 25 minutes away from a fresh, piping-hot slice of Refrigerator Pizza Dough White Pizza (page 106) than it would be to order and pick up take-out gluten-free pizza, if you're lucky enough to have that nearby. And a lot less expensive, too.

2 cups (280 g) high-quality all-purpose gluten-free flour

1½ teaspoons xanthan gum (omit if your blend already contains it)

2 teaspoons instant yeast

1 teaspoon (4 g) sugar

¾ teaspoon kosher salt

2 tablespoons (28 g) extra-virgin olive oil, plus more for drizzling

¾ cup warm water (about 100°F)

1. In a large bowl, place the flour, xanthan gum, yeast, and sugar, and whisk well with a handheld whisk. Add the salt and whisk again.

2. To the flour mixture, add the 2 tablespoons of olive oil and the water in a steady stream, mixing with a spoon or fork as you add the liquid until the mixture begins to come together. If the dough seems super sticky, add some more flour by the tablespoon, and stir to incorporate. Press the dough into a disk with well-floured hands.

3. Place the dough in another medium-size bowl and drizzle it lightly with no more than 1 tablespoon of olive oil. Turn the dough to coat it with olive oil, which will prevent a crust from forming as it rises. Cover the bowl tightly with plastic wrap.

4. If you are planning to use the dough the same day, place the dough in a warm, draft-free environment to rise until it is about 150 percent of its original volume (about 40 minutes). The dough needs to be wet (mostly with oil) when it first comes together, and as it sits—either in the refrigerator or out on the counter—the flours absorb the oils and become flexible and stable. So allow it to sit for a few minutes before rolling it out.

5. If you are not planning to use the dough the same day, place the covered bowl in the refrigerator and allow it to rise slowly for at least 12 hours and up to 4 days.

6. When you're ready to roll out the dough, remove it from the bowl and place it on a lightly floured piece of unbleached parchment paper. Cover the dough with another piece of unbleached parchment paper, and roll out until it's about ⅛ inch thick—no thinner or it will burn during baking.

7. Although pizza that has already been baked freezes quite well, for best results, do not freeze raw pizza dough.

Shoestring Savings

On a shoestring: $1.20/crust

If you bought it: $6.50/crust

very wrinkly

Yeast-Free Pizza Dough

Time Estimate: 10 minutes active time, 15 minutes inactive time

MAKES ONE 12-INCH PIZZA

Can be doubled or halved easily

....

Picture it. You're really very busy, and before you know it, it's close to dinnertime. You don't have any Yeasted Refrigerator Pizza Dough in the icebox. But you're pretty sure you have some cheese and you know you saw a jar of tomato sauce in the back of your pantry. You always have basics on hand, such as an all-purpose gluten-free flour, olive oil, and baking powder. What can you do? Here's what you can do. Use this dough in the Yeast-Free Pizza Margherita (page 110), or to replace the Yeasted Refrigerator Pizza Dough (page 63) in the White Pizza (page 106).

1½ cups (210 g) high-quality all-purpose gluten-free flour

¾ teaspoon xanthan gum (omit if your blend already contains it)

2 ¼ teaspoons baking powder

½ teaspoon kosher salt

3 tablespoons (42 g) extra-virgin olive oil

1 tablespoon honey

6 to 8 tablespoons warm water, plus more by the tablespoon if necessary

1. In a large bowl, place the flour, xanthan gum, baking powder, and salt, and whisk well.

2. Add the olive oil and honey, and mix well. It will be lumpy. Add 6 tablespoons of warm water, and mix again. Add more water by the tablespoon until the dough holds together (mostly) and isn't dry and crumbly. If you add too much water, just sprinkle in a bit of flour until the dough can be pressed together. It may be wet and tacky to the touch, but shouldn't be slick.

3. If time allows, wrap the dough in plastic wrap and allow it to sit at room temperature for 15 minutes. Then roll it out between two sheets of lightly floured unbleached parchment paper and carefully tuck it into the bottom and halfway up the sides of a nonstick or greased tart pan or cast-iron skillet for baking. If rolling it out makes the dough too difficult to handle, with wet hands, simply press it into the bottom of the pan or skillet and up the sides.

Quick-Rising Cornmeal Sandwich Bread

Time Estimate: 10 minutes active time, 1 hour 10 minutes inactive time

MAKES 1 LOAF OF BREAD

Do not double

....

This sandwich bread is dairy-free, hearty, savory, and has a nice, toothsome bite. Serve a thick slice as Texas Toast (page 48), or simply toasted with some jam.

4 tablespoons (56 g) extra-virgin olive oil, plus more for greasing loaf pan

2½ cups (350 g) high-quality all-purpose gluten-free flour

1½ teaspoons xanthan gum (omit if your blend already contains it)

1 cup (132 g) coarsely ground cornmeal

1 tablespoon instant yeast

¼ teaspoon cream of tartar

2 teaspoons kosher salt

1 teaspoon apple cider vinegar

1 teaspoon pure vanilla extract

3 tablespoons honey

1½ cups warm milk, about 100°F (low-fat is fine, nonfat is not)

1 extra-large egg plus 1 extra-large egg white, at room temperature, lightly
    beaten

1. Preheat your oven to 425°F. Grease a loaf pan that is no larger than 9 by 5 inches with olive oil and set it aside.

2. In the bowl of your stand mixer fitted with the paddle attachment, place the flour, xanthan gum, cornmeal, yeast, and cream of tartar, and whisk well with a separate handheld whisk. Add the salt and whisk again. Add the vinegar, vanilla, olive oil, honey, milk, and eggs, beating well after each addition.

3. Beat the mixture on high speed for about 5 minutes. Cover the mixer with a tea towel in case any loose bits of dough try to fly out. The dough will be thick and a bit sticky, more like batter than dough.

4. Scrape the dough with a spatula into the prepared loaf pan. Wet the spatula and smooth out the top of the dough. Cover the pan loosely with plastic wrap and

place in a warm, draft-free area to rise to a bit less than 150 percent of its original size. It is a quick-rising loaf and should only take about 25 minutes to rise just above the lip of the loaf pan.

5. Once the dough has finished rising, remove the plastic wrap. Place the pan in the center of the preheated oven and bake at 425°F for 15 minutes. Turn the oven temperature down to 375°F and slide out the oven rack to access the loaf. Wet the blade of a very sharp knife and use it to carefully make a shallow slice lengthwise down the center of the loaf, only about ¼ inch deep.

6. Return the loaf to the oven and bake for another 25 minutes. Then remove the bread from the loaf pan and place it on a rimmed baking sheet. Place the baking sheet back in the oven and finish baking the loaf until it's nicely browned on all sides and sounds hollow when tapped firmly on the side, about another 10 minutes. Remove from the oven and allow to cool before slicing.

Quick-Rising Oatmeal Molasses Bread

Time Estimate: 10 minutes active time, 1 hour 10 minutes inactive time

MAKES 1 LOAF OF BREAD

Do not double

....

Instant yeast has smaller granules than active dry yeast, which is meant to promote a faster rise. Some breads take their sweet time rising anyway, even when you use the quick stuff. This healthy and beautiful brown bread, like the Quick-Rising Cornmeal Sandwich Bread (page 66), rises as quickly as you would hope. And the smell when it's baking away in the oven is heavenly. It's better for tea than for sandwiches, but it still makes a nice strong sandwich (especially if you toast the slices).

Unsalted butter to grease loaf pan

1 cup (100 g) gluten-free old-fashioned oats, ground about halfway to flour

2¼ cups (315 g) high-quality all-purpose gluten-free flour

1½ teaspoons xanthan gum (omit if your blend already contains it)

2¼ teaspoons instant yeast

½ teaspoon cream of tartar

1 teaspoon baking soda

¼ teaspoon kosher salt

1 teaspoon apple cider vinegar

4 tablespoons (56 g) unsalted butter, at room temperature

3½ tablespoons (73 g) blackstrap molasses

1½ tablespoons Lyle's golden syrup or honey

1 extra-large egg plus 1 extra-large egg white, at room temperature, lightly beaten

1 cup milk, about 100°F (low-fat is fine, nonfat is not)

4 ounces (112 g) golden raisins tossed with ½ tablespoon (5 g) high-quality all-purpose gluten-free flour

1. Preheat your oven to 375°F. Grease a loaf pan that is no larger than 9 by 5 inches and set it aside.

2. In the bowl of your stand mixer fitted with the paddle attachment, place the ground oats, flour, xanthan gum, yeast, cream of tartar, and baking soda, and whisk well with a separate handheld whisk. Add the salt and whisk again. Add the vinegar, butter, molasses, syrup, eggs, and milk, beating well after each addition.

3. Beat the mixture on high speed for about 5 minutes. Cover the mixer with a tea towel in case any loose bits of dough try to fly out. The dough will be thick and a bit sticky.

4. Add the flour-tossed raisins and mix by hand until they are evenly distributed throughout the dough.

5. Scrape the dough with a spatula into the prepared loaf pan. Wet the spatula and smooth out the top of the dough. Cover the pan loosely with plastic wrap and place in a warm, draft-free area to rise to a bit less than 150 percent of its original size. It is a quick-rising loaf, and should only take about 25 minutes to rise just above the lip of the loaf pan.

6. Once the dough has finished rising, remove the plastic wrap. Place the pan in the center of the preheated oven. Bake for about 35 minutes. Remove the bread from the loaf pan and place it on a rimmed baking sheet. Bake the loaf another 10 minutes, until it's nicely browned on all sides and sounds hollow when tapped firmly on the side. Remove from the oven and allow to cool before slicing.

Shoestring Savings

On a shoestring: $5.50/loaf

If you bought it: $10.00/loaf

Yeasted Refrigerator Bread Dough

Time Estimate: 10 minutes active time, inactive overnight
MAKES ENOUGH FOR 12 ROLLS OR 1 LOAF OF BREAD
Do not double or halve (but you can make multiple batches serially)

Full disclosure: This is the same recipe as the White Sandwich Bread from *Gluten-Free on a Shoestring*. (Surprise!) But I'm including it again in this book because this bread dough is so wondrous, I've since discovered even more great ways to use it (see pages 72–73 and 84). Even better, the dough will keep for a week in the fridge. When I realized that I could just make some dough every Sunday and keep it on hand all week long for any number of purposes, I knew it would be perfect for *Quick and Easy*. But don't worry. It and the recipe for Flour Tortillas (page 80), which also appeared in *Gluten-Free on a Shoestring*, are bonus recipes. They don't count toward the recipe count in this book. So, technically, there are 102 recipes in this book. Jackpot, right?

(Note: This recipe doesn't double well due to the yeast, but if you need a bigger batch, just make multiple recipes of it with the same *mise en place* ingredients, using the same kitchen tools, one after the other.)

3 cups (420 g) high-quality all-purpose gluten-free flour

2 ¼ teaspoons xanthan gum (omit if your blend already contains it)

1 tablespoon instant yeast

¼ teaspoon cream of tartar

2 tablespoons sugar

2 teaspoons (25 g) kosher salt

4 tablespoons (56 g) unsalted butter, melted and cooled

1 teaspoon apple cider vinegar

2 extra-large egg whites, at room temperature

1½ cups warm milk, about 100°F (low-fat is fine, nonfat is not)

1. In the bowl of your stand mixer fitted with the paddle attachment, place the flour, xanthan gum, yeast, cream of tartar, and sugar. Whisk well with a separate handheld whisk. Add the salt and whisk again.

2. With the mixer on low speed, add the butter, cider vinegar, egg whites, and milk. Once the dry ingredients have begun to absorb the wet ingredients, mix on high speed for about 5 minutes. Cover the mixer with a tea towel to catch any loose bits of dough that may fly out of the mixing bowl. The dough should be thick and stiff, and some of it will stick to the sides of the mixing bowl.

3. Scrape the dough gently into a large resealable food-grade plastic container, one with enough room to allow it to rise to about 150 percent of its original volume. Cover, and allow to rise in the refrigerator for at least 12 hours.

4. This dough will keep in the refrigerator for up to 1 week. Do not freeze.

Boule Bread with Yeasted Refrigerator Bread Dough

Time Estimate: 10 minutes active time, 40 minutes inactive time

MAKES 1 LOAF OF BREAD

A *boule* loaf is so rustic and beautiful, it will impress the pants off your family and friends. It can be made large, with a whole recipe of dough, or divided into thirds and shaped into tapered cylinders for miniature baguettes. Simply adjust the baking time (start checking after 20 minutes) and use your imagination.

1 recipe Yeasted Refrigerator Bread Dough (page 70)

High-quality all-purpose gluten-free flour, for sprinkling and dusting

Cornstarch wash (1 tablespoon cornstarch plus ½ cup water mixed into a slurry)

    (optional; helps bread to crisp)

Toasted sesame seeds, for sprinkling (optional)

1. Preheat your oven to 400°F. If you have a pizza stone, place it on the lower rack of your oven while it is preheating. Otherwise, use an overturned rimmed baking sheet.

2. Turn out the bread dough onto a lightly floured piece of unbleached parchment paper. It will be quite sticky, even more so than when you first put it in the refrigerator. With well-floured hands, gently pat the dough into a round, 1½ to 2 inches thick, pulling the sides under the loaf where necessary to smooth the top. If your hands are sticking to the dough at all, flour them again.

3. With a very sharp knife, cut two or three ½-inch-deep slashes into the top of the loaf. With a pastry brush, cover the top of the loaf with the cornstarch wash, if using. If omitting the cornstarch wash, brush the top with milk or beaten egg whites. Sprinkle generously with the sesame seeds, if using.

4. With the bread still on the parchment paper, place it on the pizza stone or the overturned baking sheet. Spray the loaf with warm water and quickly close the oven door. Bake for about 40 minutes, or until deep golden brown and crusty. Rotate once during baking, and periodically spray the loaf with warm water.

5. Remove from the oven and place on a wire rack to cool completely before slicing and serving.

Dinner Rolls with Yeasted Refrigerator Bread Dough

Time Estimate: 10 minutes active time, 25 minutes inactive time

MAKES 12 ROLLS

I told you that this Yeasted Refrigerator Bread Dough (page 70) was versatile. Dinner rolls are ready so fast, with no resting, no second rise, and no planning beyond what you did over the weekend to make that dough. You know it's your dinner-finishing ace in the hole.

1 recipe Yeasted Refrigerator Bread Dough (page 70)
High-quality all-purpose gluten-free flour, for sprinkling and dusting
Cornstarch wash (1 tablespoon cornstarch plus ½ cup water mixed into a slurry)
    (optional; helps bread to crisp)

1. Preheat your oven to 400°F. If you have a pizza stone, place it on the lower rack of your oven while it is preheating. Otherwise, use an overturned rimmed baking sheet. Line a separate rimmed baking sheet with unbleached parchment paper and set it aside.

2. Turn out the bread dough onto a lightly floured piece of unbleached parchment paper. It will be quite sticky, even more so than when you first put it in the refrigerator. With well-floured hands, pat the dough into a rectangle. With a well-floured bench scraper or sharp knife, divide the dough into twelve pieces. With well-floured hands, shape each piece of dough gently into a round, stretching the dough across the top of the round and tucking it underneath for a smooth top.

3. Place the rolls about an inch apart on the prepared baking sheet. With a pastry brush, cover the top of each roll with the cornstarch wash (if using). If omitting the cornstarch wash, brush the tops with milk or beaten egg whites.

4. Place the baking sheet in the center of the preheated oven, on top of the pizza stone or on top of the overturned baking sheet. Bake for about 25 minutes, or until the rolls are golden brown, rotating once during baking.

5. Remove the rolls from the oven and place on a wire rack to cool completely before serving.

Shoestring Savings

On a shoestring: 48¢ each

If you bought it: $1.00 each

Saltine-Style Crackers

Time Estimate: 25 minutes
MAKES ABOUT 20 CRACKERS, DEPENDING UPON SIZE
Can be doubled or halved

··

These little ditties are so simple, but the ingredient balance has to be just right or they, well, won't be. So portion your ingredients carefully, and be sure each is of good quality. The flour especially shines through in such a simple cracker.

1 cup plus 2 tablespoons (156 g) high-quality all-purpose gluten-free flour

½ teaspoon xanthan gum (omit if your blend already contains it)

¼ teaspoon baking soda

1¼ teaspoons baking powder

1 tablespoon granulated sugar

¼ teaspoon kosher salt, plus extra for dusting

¼ teaspoon cream of tartar

2 tablespoons (24 g) vegetable shortening

1 tablespoon (14 g) unsalted butter, at room temperature

⅓ cup water, at room temperature, plus more by the tablespoon if necessary

1. Preheat your oven to 350°F. Line a rimmed baking sheet with unbleached parchment paper and set it aside.

2. In the bowl of your food processor fitted with the metal blade, place the flour, xanthan gum, baking soda, baking powder, sugar, ¼ teaspoon of the salt, and the cream of tartar, and pulse a few times to mix well.

3. Add the shortening and butter, and pulse until the mixture is sandy in texture. With the food processor running, add the water a tablespoon at a time. Once all the water has gone in, turn off the machine and pulse once quickly. The dough should be soft and shiny, but not very wet. If the dough is smooth and integrated, dump it out onto an unbleached parchment paper–lined countertop. If it seems a bit too wet, add more flour by the teaspoon and pulse. If it seems too dry, add a tablespoon of water and pulse.

4. With lightly floured hands, gather the dough together and pat it into a rectangle. Place another sheet of unbleached parchment paper on top, and roll out the dough to about ¼ inch thick. With a pastry wheel, slice it into rectangles that are about 1½ by 2½ inches.

5. With a floured offset (or angled) spatula, transfer the rectangles to the prepared baking sheet, arranging less than an inch apart. They won't spread during baking. Pierce each cracker a few times with the tines of a fork. With wet fingers, lightly moisten the top of each cracker. Sprinkle evenly with kosher salt, to taste.

6. Place the baking sheet in the center of the preheated oven and bake, rotating once during baking, for about 8 minutes, or until the cracker edges are just beginning to brown. Allow them to cool briefly on the baking sheet until firm.

7. Serve immediately. Wrap leftovers loosely in waxed paper and store at room temperature for a day or so. But I doubt there will be too many leftovers.

Shoestring Savings

On a shoestring: 7¢ each or 80¢ for 12

If you bought it: 26¢ each or $3.00 for 12

Goldfish-Style Crackers

Time Estimate: 30 minutes

MAKES ABOUT 4 DOZEN CRACKERS, DEPENDING UPON SIZE

Can be doubled or halved easily

So cute! Schär makes some nice crackers for the little ones, but they're not fish-shaped. They're probably not allowed to be. But we can do whatever we like! If it's a fish-shaped cookie cutter you're seeking, you can buy one online at CopperGifts.com (search for "mini goldfish"). I was way too cheap to shell out the required $8 plus shipping, so I sacrificed a relatively small heart-shaped cookie cutter I already had, and bent it to my will. Then, I made most of my fish with happy faces, but I made a few grumpy. With mean eyebrows and everything. I'm not always so chipper, you know. Are you?

1 cup (140 g) high-quality all-purpose gluten-free flour

½ teaspoon xanthan gum (omit if your blend already contains it)

½ teaspoon kosher salt

Dash (⅛ teaspoon) of baking soda

½ teaspoon smoked Spanish paprika

4 tablespoons (48 g) vegetable shortening

10 ounces Kraft Velveeta cheese

2 to 4 tablespoons ice water

1. Preheat your oven to 350°F. Line rimmed baking sheets with unbleached parchment paper and set them aside.

2. In the bowl of your food processor fitted with the steel blade, place the flour, xanthan gum, salt, baking soda, and paprika. Pulse a few times to mix the dry ingredients. Cut the shortening and Velveeta roughly into pieces and add them to the bowl. Cover and pulse a few times until the mixture resembles crumbs.

3. Add 2 tablespoons of water and pulse a few times. If the mixture doesn't begin to come together, add another tablespoon of water and pulse again a few times. Repeat with the remaining tablespoon of water if necessary. The dough should begin to come away from the walls of the food processor.

4. Turn out the dough onto a piece of unbleached parchment paper. Divide the dough in half and set one portion aside. Cover the remaining half with another piece of unbleached parchment paper and roll it out until it is about ¼ inch thick. Use a small fish-shaped cookie cutter to cut out fish shapes. Place them less than an inch apart on the prepared baking sheets. Gather the scraps and reroll. Repeat with the remaining dough.

5. To make happy fish, use the tapered point of a #1 or #2 pastry tip to create an eye, and the wide end to press a half-moon smile into each fish.

6. Bake the crackers in the center of the oven for 8 to 10 minutes, or until just beginning to brown around the edges, rotating the sheet once during baking. Remove the baking sheet from the oven, and allow the crackers to cool briefly until firm.

7. Store any leftovers in a sealed container at room temperature for a day or so.

Shoestring Savings

**On a shoestring: 8¢ each,
or $1.60 for 20**

**If you bought it: 14¢ each,
or $2.80 for 20**

Pan de Bono

Time Estimate: 10 minutes active time, 20 minutes inactive time

MAKES 8 TO 10 ROLLS

Can be halved easily, but not doubled
unless you have a 14-cup food processor

....

This is similar to Brazilian cheese bread, which is much chewier and made without benefit of the lovely and talented masa harina, a precooked cornmeal. *Pan de bono* is a naturally gluten-free Colombian bread that's as versatile as it is flavorful. The dough is easy to handle when prepared precisely according to the instructions. If you are having any trouble, refrigerate the dough for a bit and try again. The dough itself also freezes surprisingly well. Just thaw in the refrigerator and proceed with the rest of the recipe.

8 ounces queso fresco (Mexican), quesito (Colombian), or feta cheese (Greek)

⅓ cup (39 g) gluten-free masa harina

⅔ cup (80 g) gluten-free tapioca starch (also called tapioca flour)

½ teaspoon kosher salt

1 extra-large egg, at room temperature, beaten

2 tablespoons (28 g) unsalted butter, melted

1. Preheat your oven to 375°F. Line a rimmed baking sheet with unbleached parchment paper and set it aside.

2. Place the cheese in the bowl of a food processor and pulse until all the large pieces are crumbled into uniformly pebble-size pieces. Add the masa harina, tapioca starch, and salt, and pulse until well mixed.

3. With the food processor on, add the egg and blend until a very smooth, integrated ball forms (about 2 minutes). You might have to stop the food processor halfway through to scrape down the sides of the bowl.

4. Turn the dough onto a piece of plastic wrap on the counter, press into a disk, and wrap tightly. Place the dough in the freezer for 5 to 10 minutes, or until firm.

5. Once the dough has chilled, divide it into eight or ten pieces (larger pieces and fewer of them, if you prefer), roll them into balls, and place about 1 inch apart on the prepared baking sheet.

6. Place in the center of the preheated oven, and bake for about 15 to 20 minutes, or until lightly browned on top, rotating once during baking. Right before you remove the rolls from the oven, pierce a hole in the top of each to allow steam to escape and the rolls to keep their shape.

7. Remove the rolls from the oven, brush generously with the melted butter, and allow to cool before serving.

Flour Tortillas

Time Estimate: 20 minutes

MAKES 6 TORTILLAS

Can be doubled or halved easily

....

This recipe is also included in *Gluten-Free on a Shoestring*, but flour tortillas are so essential to the proper working of a weekday gluten-free kitchen that I wanted to make absolutely sure that you have them at your fingertips.

Of course, you can always substitute corn tortillas in any recipe that calls for flour tortillas, but once you get the hang of making this recipe, you will see how you can dream up Beef and Cheese Burritos (page 143) and have them on the table in 35 minutes flat, fresh flour tortillas and all.

2 cups (280 g) high-quality all-purpose gluten-free flour

1 teaspoon xanthan gum (omit if your blend already contains it)

1½ teaspoons baking powder

1 teaspoon kosher salt

4 teaspoons (19 g) neutral oil (like canola or grapeseed)

¾ to 1 cup water, at room temperature

1. In a large bowl, place the flour, xanthan gum, baking powder, and salt, and whisk well. Create a well in the center and add the oil and ¾ cup of water, and stir to incorporate.

2. The mixture should begin to come together. Add more water by the tablespoon if the dough is at all crumbly. It should hold together and be a bit tacky to the touch, but not sticky.

3. Divide the dough into six equal pieces. Take a gallon-size resealable plastic bag, cut off the zip-top, and slice the bag into two equal pieces by cutting along the two seams and then along the bottom seam. If you have a tortilla press, prepare a quart-size resealable plastic bag in the same way, and use it to line the tortilla press. Flatten each piece of dough in the press, and then place it between the two pieces of plastic from the gallon-size bag.

4. Roll each piece of dough between the two pieces of plastic from the gallon-size bag (whether you have used a tortilla press or not) until the dough is about ⅛ inch thick (the thickness of a nickel) and about 8 inches wide. Do not roll it too thin, or it will be too difficult to handle. If the rolled-out dough breaks when you attempt to remove it from the plastic, it is too wet. Add more flour by the tablespoon, and knead it to incorporate it into the dough.

5. Heat a large cast-iron or nonstick skillet over medium-high heat. Once the skillet is hot, place a raw tortilla flat in the skillet, one at a time. Allow each to cook for 45 to 60 seconds, or until it begins to bubble, taking care not to burn the tortilla or it won't be pliable.

6. With a large, heatproof spatula, flip the tortilla and cook for another 30 to 45 seconds, remove from the pan, and wrap in a moist tea towel.

7. These are best used when they're still warm. Fill them while they're still warm, wrap them in plastic wrap, and unwrap and heat when ready to eat.

Shoestring Savings

On a shoestring: 36¢ each

If you bought it: $1.16 each

Quick Puff Pastry

Time Estimate: 20 minutes active time, 1 hour 10 minutes inactive time

MAKES 6 SERVINGS

Can be doubled easily

....

When I say "quick" here, I mean "quicker." If you want puffy pastry, it's going to eat up a bit of time. This method starts with clumps of butter, rather than a one-pound block of it. You sacrifice a wee bit of the puffiness, but not too much.

The "turns" associated with puff pastry are outlined, in step-by-step photographic splendor, on my blog in the recipe for Traditional Puff Pastry (http://gluten freeonashoestring.com/gluten-free-puff-pastry-with-better-batter/). The general idea of these turns is that they create alternating layers of pastry dough and large chunks of butter. As the dough is rolled out and then folded over on itself, more layers are formed. When the cold butter hits the hot oven, it expands and pushes out the layers of dough, creating a puffy and flaky pastry. If this is new to you, read the recipe a few times before you do a thing, then give it a try. It really does work, and when it does, it's very exciting indeed.

2 ¼ cups (315 g) high-quality all-purpose gluten-free flour

1 teaspoon xanthan gum (omit if your blend already contains it)

½ teaspoon kosher salt

16 tablespoons (224 g) unsalted butter, cut into tablespoons and
    kept refrigerated

¼ to ½ cup water, iced (ice cubes don't count in volume measurement)

1. In a large bowl, whisk together the flour, xanthan gum, and salt. Take one stick's worth of butter (8 tablespoons). Flatten each tablespoon of butter between your fingers and then add it to the dry ingredients, mixing to distribute the butter evenly. Add ¼ cup of the ice water to the bowl, and mix carefully just to combine the flour and butter. Add more water, 1 tablespoon at a time, until the dough holds loosely together.

2. Turn out the dough onto a piece of unbleached parchment paper. With well-floured hands, shape it into a ½-inch-thick rectangle. Cover the rectangle tightly with plastic wrap and freeze until firm but not frozen solid, about 10 minutes.

3. Once the dough has chilled, remove the plastic wrap, then press and roll out the dough between two pieces of unbleached parchment paper into a roughly 10 by 15-inch rectangle that is about ¼ inch thick, no thinner. Remove the top sheet of parchment paper. Dust the dough with additional flour as necessary to prevent it from sticking to the parchment paper. Take the remaining 8 tablespoons of chilled butter and space them evenly over two-thirds of the dough, leaving one short side bare. With the bare, short side facing you, fold it over the middle third of the butter (as you would a business letter), then fold the remaining third over to seal in the tablespoons of butter.

4. Replace the top parchment. With a short side of the dough facing your body, roll the dough away from you into a rectangle about 10 by 15 inches. Fold again in thirds as you would a business letter. Cover with plastic wrap and place in the freezer for 10 minutes, or until firm. Congratulations. You have just completed the first pastry "turn."

5. Remove the dough from the freezer, uncover it, and place it horizontally on a fresh sheet of unbleached parchment paper. Cover with another sheet of unbleached parchment paper. With a short side again facing your body, roll away from you into a rectangle about 10 by 15 inches. Fold once more, business letter style, and return to the freezer for another 10 minutes or until firm. Repeat the process once more. After four turns, cover and place the dough in the freezer for about 10 minutes, until firm.

6. To use, roll out the dough again into a smaller rectangle about ⅜ inch thick. Slice and use however you like.

7. Fold any remaining dough in thirds and wrap tightly in plastic wrap. Place in a freezer-safe resealable plastic bag, and freeze until ready to use. Before using frozen puff pastry, allow it to thaw a bit in the refrigerator for an hour.

SUGGESTIONS FOR USE: Use to top the Quick Chicken Pot Pie (page 132); use in place of regular pastry dough for a pie; score the perimeter of the dough with a sharp knife, top the center with thin pear slices, sprinkle with cinnamon and sugar, and bake at 350°F for 15 minutes, or until nicely browned and flaky; cut rounds, brush with milk, sprinkle with sugar, and bake at 350°F for 10 minutes, or until nicely browned and flaky.

Garlic Parmesan Breadsticks

Time Estimate: 15 minutes active time, 15 minutes inactive time
MAKES 12 BREADSTICKS

....

For good measure, here are breadsticks made with the now-famous Yeasted Refrigerator Bread Dough (page 70). Don't like garlic? Leave it out. Unless I'm coming
to dinner. Then make a few for me with garlic, and just don't plan to kiss me when
the night is through. Okay, fine. Kiss me, you fool.

1 recipe Yeasted Refrigerator Bread Dough (page 70)
High-quality all-purpose gluten-free flour, for sprinkling and dusting
3 tablespoons unsalted butter, melted
¼ teaspoon garlic salt
¼ cup finely grated Parmigiano-Reggiano
Kosher salt, for sprinkling

1. Preheat your oven to 400°F. Place a pizza stone (or overturned rimmed baking sheet) on the lower rack of your oven while it is preheating. Line a separate
rimmed baking sheet with unbleached parchment paper and set it aside.

2. Turn out the bread dough onto a lightly floured piece of unbleached parchment paper. It will be quite sticky, even more so than when you first put it in the
refrigerator. With well-floured hands, pat the dough into a rectangle. With a well-
floured bench scraper or sharp knife, divide the dough into twelve pieces.

3. With well-floured hands, roll each piece of dough back and forth to form a
6-inch cylinder. Place the breadsticks about 2 inches apart on the prepared baking
sheet.

4. Place the melted butter, garlic salt, and grated cheese in a small bowl, and
mix well. Brush the pieces of dough with the melted butter mixture and sprinkle
lightly with kosher salt.

5. Place the baking sheet in the center of the preheated oven, on top of the
pizza stone or on the overturned rimmed baking sheet. Bake for about 15 minutes, or until the breadsticks are light golden brown, rotating once during baking.
Allow to cool before serving.

Basic Pastry Crust

Time Estimate: 10 minutes active time, 15 minutes inactive time
MAKES ENOUGH CRUST FOR A TOP AND BOTTOM OF A PIE
Can be doubled or halved easily

Because this dough is not yeasted, it freezes well. I highly recommend making some pastry crust and keeping it on hand for recipes such as Quick Chicken Pot Pie (page 132). It will keep for 3 to 4 days quite nicely in the refrigerator, and longer than that in the freezer. If you're freezing it, just be sure to divide it into portions and wrap well in a freezer-safe wrap, and then in a freezer-safe resealable plastic bag. Thaw overnight in the refrigerator before using.

TIP: If you're afraid to make and roll out pastry crust, I've got you covered. I did a how-to video that you can find on YouTube. Just search "Nicloe Hunn pastry crust," or go directly to http://www.youtube.com/watch?v=BXLszvOxhmk.

2¼ cups (315 g) high-quality all-purpose gluten-free flour

1 teaspoon xanthan gum (omit if your blend already contains it)

½ teaspoon baking powder

½ teaspoon kosher salt

10 tablespoons (140 g) unsalted butter, chopped roughly and chilled

½ to ¾ cup water, iced (ice cubes don't count in the volume measurement)

1. In a large bowl, place the flour, xanthan gum, baking powder, and salt. Whisk the dry ingredients until well combined. Add the chunks of butter and flatten each chunk with well-floured fingers.

2. Add ½ cup of ice water to the mixture a bit at a time, mixing to combine. After you have added this first ½ cup of ice water, if the mixture has not yet come together, drizzle in more water by the scant tablespoon and mix. Stop adding water the moment the mixture begins to come together.

3. Turn out the dough onto a large sheet of plastic wrap, enclose lightly, and place in the freezer until firm, about 15 minutes. If you are not planning to use the dough right away, transfer the wrapped dough to the refrigerator, where it can keep for a few days. Otherwise, freeze until solid and thaw in the refrigerator overnight before using.

Chapter 5

··

Meatless Mondays

(OR, VEGGIES EVEN MY PICKIEST KID MIGHT EAT)

love animals. I rescue cute little furry animals. I also eat animals.
For many years, I didn't eat any animals. And then I started having children, and they were hungry. The end.

That isn't to say, however, that I don't love my vegetables. I do, and I always have. I never ventured too far into veganism, because I missed real cheese too much. But I consider eating vegetables to be an essential part of life. Lucky for me, two of my three children agree. The third is a much harder sell, but she's much more compliant when the vegetables are in *stromboli*, or pressed into a black bean veggie burger or falafel. I don't hide the vegetables, but I'm not above commingling them to make them taste too good to resist.

- 🐾 Mushroom and Spinach Stromboli
- 🐾 Baked Egg Dinner
- 🐾 Veggie Burgers
- 🐾 Black Bean and Spinach Burritos
- 🐾 Pressure Cooker Scratch Black Beans
- 🐾 Vegetable Clafouti
- 🐾 Quick Vegetable Paella

- Polenta Bake
- Egg Fried Rice
- Baked Falafel
- Refrigerator Pizza Dough White Pizza
- Vegetable Calzones
- Yeast-Free Pizza Margherita
- Vegetarian Chili
- Tomato and Corn Risotto

Mushroom and Spinach Stromboli

SERVES 4

Time Estimate: 15 minutes active time, 20 minutes inactive time

Can be doubled or halved easily

....

Stromboli is like pizza—the varieties are infinite, and as long as there's cheese, you aren't likely to hear anyone complaining at the dinner table. Feel free to replace the spinach with another leafy green such as kale, or something different, such as blanched and drained broccoli florets. Whichever way you go, with that Yeasted Refrigerator Pizza Dough, it's a quick and satisfying weekday meal.

1 recipe Yeasted Refrigerator Pizza Dough (page 63)

2 to 4 tablespoons extra-virgin olive oil, plus more for brushing

1 medium-size yellow onion, peeled and diced

2 cloves garlic, smashed and peeled

8 ounces mushrooms, sliced (I like baby portobello, but any kind will do)

1 (1-pound) bag fresh, triple-washed baby spinach

Kosher salt and freshly ground black pepper

8 to 10 ounces freshly grated mozzarella cheese

1. Preheat your oven to 425°F. Place a pizza stone (or an overturned rimmed baking sheet if you don't have one) in the oven as it heats.

2. Divide the pizza dough into two portions. Roll out each between two sheets of unbleached parchment paper into a rectangle about ⅛ inch thick (no thinner; thicker if you prefer). Set the dough aside.

3. In a heavy-bottomed skillet, place 2 tablespoons of the olive oil, the diced onion, and the smashed and peeled garlic cloves. Cook the onion and garlic in the oil over medium-high heat, stirring frequently, until the onion is translucent and the garlic is fragrant (about 6 minutes). Add the sliced mushrooms and stir. Add the other 2 tablespoons of olive oil if the pan is starting to look a bit dry.

4. Turn down the heat to medium-low and cover the skillet. Cook, shaking the pan if the mushrooms begin to stick and lifting the lid to stir occasionally, until the mushrooms are softened and cooked through (about 5 minutes).

5. Add the spinach and stir. Replace the lid and cook until the spinach is mostly wilted, about another minute. Uncover the pan, season with salt and pepper to taste, and set the mixture aside to cool a bit.

6. Divide the filling between both pieces of pizza dough, leaving a 1-inch border on both long sides of the rectangle, and a 2-inch border along the short sides. Cover each with half of the grated cheese. Moisten the border of one short side with water. Starting on the other short side, which should be nearest you, roll the dough away from you as tightly as you can. Repeat with the other rectangle. Brush the tops and sides of both generously with olive oil.

7. Place both *stromboli* on a piece of unbleached parchment paper and then on the pizza stone or the overturned rimmed baking sheet. Bake for about 20 minutes, or until they are well browned and the cheese is melted and bubbling. Serve warm.

Shoestring Savings

On a shoestring: $2.81/serving

If you bought it: $5.95/serving (frozen)

Baked Egg Dinner

MAKES 4 SERVINGS
Time Estimate: 5 minutes active time, 31 minutes inactive time
Can be doubled or halved easily

....

Not too many people eat eggs for breakfast any more. Do they? Either way, it seems fitting for eggs to replace meat as a protein for your evening meal. In this recipe, the eggs bake and the cheese browns as the stock and tomato sauce cook the dried pasta and create a nice, thick sauce, all at the same time. The recipe only takes about 35 minutes, total, and most of it is inactive time because you don't even have to precook the pasta.

12 ounces short gluten-free dried pasta (such as fusilli)
1 cup tomato sauce
2 cups vegetable stock
10 ounces freshly grated mozzarella cheese
4 extra-large eggs
½ cup finely grated Parmigiano-Reggiano cheese

1. Preheat your oven to 400°F. Lightly oil four round, oven-safe crocks or soup bowls, each of 10- to 12-ounce capacity. Place them on a rimmed baking sheet and set them aside.

2. In each crock, place 3 ounces of dried pasta (one-quarter of the whole amount). Cover with ¼ cup of tomato sauce and ½ cup of stock. Mix gently. Divide the grated mozzarella cheese evenly among the top of the mixture in each crock. Crack an egg on top of the cheese in each crock, and sprinkle evenly with Parmigiano-Reggiano cheese.

3. Cover each crock with aluminum foil, making sure you don't press the foil against the cheese or it will stick as it melts. Place the rimmed baking sheet in the center of oven. Bake for about 25 minutes, until the pasta is al dente and the egg white is opaque. Uncover the crocks and bake until the cheese is nicely browned, about another 6 minutes. Serve warm.

Veggie Burgers

MAKES 4 TO 6 BURGERS, DEPENDING UPON SIZE
Time Estimate: 40 minutes
Can be doubled or halved easily

....

You can make these black bean burgers without the cooked onion, potatoes, carrots, and celery, but they just won't be as flavorful. If you really want to make quick work of these burgers, make the mixture ahead of time, form the patties, and allow them to chill in the refrigerator during the day. When you come home, all that's left to do is sauté the burgers and finish baking the rolls—and a satisfying dinner is on the table in mere minutes.

1 medium-size yellow onion, peeled and diced

2 medium-size potatoes, chopped with the skin on

2 medium-size carrots, peeled and chopped

2 celery stalks, chopped

6 to 8 tablespoons extra-virgin olive oil

1 tablespoon ground cumin

¼ teaspoon Mexican chili powder

Kosher salt and freshly ground black pepper

2 cups cooked black beans or 1 (15-ounce) can, drained and rinsed

½ cup (50 g) gluten-free old-fashioned rolled oats

5 egg yolks (large or extra-large will do)

¾ cup (105 g) high-quality all-purpose gluten-free flour, plus more for dusting

⅓ teaspoon xanthan gum (omit if your blend already contains it)

4 Schär Ciabatta Parbaked Rolls

1. In a large, heavy-bottomed saucepan, place the onion, potatoes, carrots, and celery in 3 to 4 tablespoons of oil. Stir, and turn the heat to medium-high. Add the cumin, chili powder, and salt and pepper to taste, and stir. Cover the pot and cook, stirring occasionally, to caramelize the onion and soften the vegetables, about 10 minutes.

2. While the vegetables are cooking, combine the beans, oats, and egg yolks in a food processor and pulse until the mixture is uniformly chunky but not a puree.

3. Once the vegetables are done cooking, mash them with a potato masher or fork until mashed but chunky. Allow them to cool briefly to avoid cooking the egg yolks in the black bean mixture once everything is combined.

4. Add one-third of the black bean mixture to the mashed vegetables, and stir. Add the remaining black bean mixture and stir in the flour and xanthan gum. The mixture should be very thick and you should be able to handle it enough to gently form it into patties. If you can't, add more flour by the tablespoon until you can.

5. Dredge the patties through a bit more flour and sauté them in the remaining oil over medium-high heat. Work in batches if necessary to avoid crowding, and sauté until crispy on the outside, 3 to 4 minutes per side. Transfer to plates lined with paper towels.

6. Finish baking the ciabatta buns according to the package directions. I like to bake them in a toaster oven so I don't have to wait for my conventional oven to preheat. Serve the black bean burgers warm, on a bun.

Shoestring Savings

On a shoestring: 92¢ each

If you bought it: $2.25 each (frozen)

Black Bean and Spinach Burritos

MAKES 4 TO 6 SERVINGS

Time Estimate: 35 minutes active time, including making Flour Tortillas
(see page 80)

Can be doubled or halved easily

....

This is one of those recipes that you will make faster and faster each time. Then, one day, you'll be a flour-tortilla-and-burrito-making ninja, and you'll come to rely upon those skills when the chips are down: It's your turn to drive the carpool and you have no meat in the house. I keep a rotating supply of these burritos in my freezer at all times, for when I'm really caught with my big girl pants down.

1 medium-size onion, peeled and diced

2 cloves garlic, smashed and peeled

3 tablespoons extra-virgin olive oil

1 teaspoon ground cumin

½ teaspoon Mexican chili powder, or to taste

Kosher salt and freshly ground black pepper

3 cups leftover cooked brown rice (chilled works best)

1 (15-ounce) can black beans, drained and rinsed

½ cup mild prepared salsa

1 (1-pound) bag fresh triple-washed baby spinach

8 Flour Tortillas (page 80), kept warm, or 8 corn tortillas, moistened and warmed
    in the microwave oven until pliable

6 to 8 ounces Monterey Jack cheese, grated

½ cup sour cream

1. In a large skillet, sauté the onion and garlic in the oil over medium-high heat, stirring frequently, until the onion is translucent and the garlic is fragrant, about 6 minutes. Add the cumin, chili powder, and salt and pepper to taste, and stir. Add the rice, beans, and salsa and stir, taking care not to smash the beans. Lower the heat to medium and cook until heated through.

2. Place the spinach in a separate skillet and add a splash of water. Cover and cook over medium-high heat until just wilted, about 1 minute. Remove from the heat.

3. Open the first tortilla, sprinkle a bit of cheese, and then spoon about one-sixth of the rice mixture across the center of the tortilla. Top with some wilted spinach, more grated cheese, and a dollop of sour cream. Fold in the sides of the tortilla, and roll away from you until the tortilla is sealed. Press down lightly.

4. Repeat with the remaining tortillas. Microwave each tortilla on HIGH for about 45 seconds, or until the cheese is fully melted and has sealed the burrito closed. Allow to cool briefly before serving. This will allow the burrito to become firm enough to handle.

Shoestring Savings

On a shoestring: $1.56 each

If you bought it: $3.84 each (frozen)

Pressure Cooker Scratch Black Beans

MAKES ABOUT 6 CUPS COOKED BLACK BEANS

Time Estimate: 15 minutes active time, 25 minutes inactive time

Can be halved easily (not doubled unless your pressure cooker is ginormous)

....

If you're among the uninitiated, allow me to introduce you to the wonders of pressure cooking. I've never been much of a slow-cooker sort of person. I'm fast! I'm better on the fly. And because I'm not that much of a planner, my pressure cooker has rescued me on many a weeknight.

If you're at all concerned about the safety of pressure cookers, know that they've come a long way since the time when they would explode if you weren't lucky. These days, they regulate pressure by allowing some to escape during cooking, when necessary. You don't have to do a thing more than toss in the ingredients, bring it to pressure over a high flame, lower the heat to medium, and wait the prescribed amount of time.

This recipe assumes that you have not soaked the beans. If you choose to soak them first, simply cut the cooking time by 10 minutes. Add vegetable stock and a jar of prepared salsa to the beans, and you have black bean soup. Serve with some crusty bread for a complete meal.

6 tablespoons extra-virgin olive oil

2 medium-size yellow onions, peeled and diced

6 cloves garlic, smashed and peeled

1 pound dried black beans, rinsed

4 cups vegetable stock

4 cups water

Kosher salt and freshly ground black pepper

1. In a pressure cooker with at least a 6-quart capacity, place 4 tablespoons of the olive oil, the diced onions, and the garlic. Cook over medium-high heat without the cover, stirring frequently, until the onions are translucent and the garlic is fragrant, about 6 minutes. Add the black beans and the remaining 2 tablespoons of oil, and stir to mix and coat the beans with oil.

2. Add the stock and water, then cover the pressure cooker and lock its lid in place. Allow everything to cook over high heat until the button pops, letting you know it has reached pressure at 15 psi. Turn down the heat to medium and cook for 25 minutes. Remove the pot from the heat and allow it to reduce pressure naturally. Once the pressure is reduced, the pressure button will depress on its own. Once it does, carefully remove the lid.

3. Drain off the remaining liquid into a separate container for later use (see headnote for serving suggestions). Season to taste with salt and pepper.

Vegetable Clafouti

MAKES 4 SERVINGS

Time Estimate: 15 minutes active time, 20 minutes inactive time

Can be doubled or halved easily

....

It's amazing what cream and eggs can do to put a meal on the table in no time, especially when you mix them with some savory vegetables and cheese. Although I wouldn't consider this meal something I'd eat every day, as it is rather decadent, it sure makes for a nice change of pace.

Unsalted butter for greasing ramekins

1 medium-size yellow onion, peeled and diced

3 tablespoons extra-virgin olive oil

1 large or 2 small yellow summer squash, chopped

1 pound grape or cherry tomatoes, sliced in half

½ cup finely grated Parmigiano-Romano cheese

6 ounces fresh mozzarella cheese, cut into ½-inch cubes

1 large handful fresh basil, chopped roughly

1 large handful fresh parsley, chopped roughly

½ cup plus 1 tablespoon (79 g) high-quality all-purpose gluten-free flour

¼ teaspoon xanthan gum (omit if your blend already contains it)

Kosher salt and freshly ground black pepper

4 extra-large eggs, at room temperature, lightly beaten

2 cups heavy whipping cream, at room temperature

1. Preheat your oven to 400°F. Grease well four 1-cup ramekins (or one 4- to 6-cup ramekin) with unsalted butter and set them aside.

2. In a large skillet over medium heat, cook the onion in the olive oil, stirring frequently, for about 6 minutes, or until softened. Add the squash and tomatoes, and cook, still stirring frequently, until the vegetables have begun to release their liquid, 4 to 5 minutes. Remove from the heat and set aside to cool briefly.

3. In a large bowl, place the Parmesan, mozzarella, basil, parsley, flour, xanthan gum, salt, and pepper, and mix until just combined. Add the eggs and cream, and then the vegetable mixture, and stir gently but fully.

4. Divide the batter evenly among the prepared ramekins. Place all four ramekins on a large rimmed baking sheet and place in the center of the preheated oven. Bake until puffed and light golden brown on top, about 20 minutes. Serve warm.

Quick Vegetable Paella

MAKES 4 SERVINGS

Time Estimate: 20 minutes active time, 20 minutes inactive time

Can be doubled or halved easily

....

The essence of paella is that the short-grain rice cooks without being stirred, and crisps on the bottom as it finishes cooking in the oven. Saffron adds some nice depth of flavor, especially in vegetable paella, which doesn't have as many competing flavors as do some other paella varieties. While the saffron isn't essential and can be expensive, a little does go a long way.

If you've ever been intimidated by paella, because of the saffron or for any other reason, let go of all that. It doesn't need elaborate ingredients to be special. To speed things up, these directions call for heating the stock in the microwave, rather than on the stovetop. Warming the stock allows it to be absorbed more easily by the rice.

4 cups vegetable stock

Pinch of saffron threads, about 12 threads (optional)

4 tablespoons extra-virgin olive oil

1 medium-size onion, peeled and diced

2 cloves garlic, peeled and smashed

1 large sweet pepper (green, red, or yellow), seeded and diced

14 ounces (half a 28-ounce can) whole peeled tomatoes, drained and chopped
     roughly

1 tablespoon tomato paste

¾ teaspoon smoked Spanish paprika

2½ cups uncooked Arborio rice (or other short-grain rice)

Kosher salt and freshly ground black pepper

1. Preheat your oven to 400°F.

2. In a large, microwave-safe bowl, place the vegetable stock and saffron threads (if using). Cover with plastic wrap and set the bowl aside.

3. In a large, oven-safe skillet (if you have a paella pan, use it; if not, a cast-iron or stainless-steel skillet works great—surface area is what we're going for), heat the olive oil over medium heat. Sauté the onion and garlic, stirring frequently, until the onion is translucent and the garlic is fragrant, about 6 minutes. Add the diced pepper and tomatoes, and cook for another 3 minutes, until the peppers begin to soften. Add the tomato paste, paprika, and rice, and stir. Cook, stirring frequently, until the rice begins to become translucent, about 5 minutes.

4. Place the large bowl of stock in the microwave and heat on HIGH for 2 minutes, or until very warm. Add the broth to the skillet and stir until just incorporated. Add salt and pepper to taste.

5. Bake the paella in the center of the oven, uncovered, for about 20 minutes, or until the rice has absorbed the liquid and is beginning to crisp on the bottom. Serve hot or warm.

Polenta Bake

MAKES 4 SERVINGS

Time Estimate: 15 minutes active time, 5 minutes inactive time

Can be doubled or halved easily

....

This quick-cooking polenta makes a warm and comforting side dish for a meal, but for my family it can even take center stage when it's broiled instead of served smooth. Feel free to leave out the cherry tomatoes before broiling and replace them with something else you love, such as salty pitted and brined olives. If you don't care for olives, please forgive my lapse in reason in suggesting them. Olives tend to evoke strong emotions, both pro and con (I'm pro, my very wrong family is con).

3 cups vegetable stock
3 tablespoons (42 g) unsalted butter
Kosher salt and freshly ground black pepper
1 cup (170 g) De la Estancia organic polenta
1 cup (80 g) finely grated Parmigiano-Reggiano
¾ cup (188 g) ricotta cheese
1 pint (2 cups) cherry tomatoes, halved

1. Place the stock, butter, and salt and pepper to taste in a medium-size, oven-proof skillet. Bring the mixture to a boil over medium-high heat.

2. Turn down the heat to medium-low and gradually stir in the polenta. Cook, stirring constantly, for 1 minute, or until thickened and beginning to pull away from the sides of the skillet. Sprinkle on the Parmesan evenly and place the ricotta cheese in dollops about an inch apart. Scatter the tomatoes on top.

3. Turn on your oven's broiler and place the skillet 4 inches away from the flame. Broil for about 5 minutes, or until golden. Serve immediately.

Egg Fried Rice

MAKES 4 SERVINGS

Time Estimate: 20 minutes active time

Can be doubled or halved easily

···

The secret to fried rice, as I understand it, is to use the proper rice. It shouldn't be newly cooked, it must be cold, and it must not have been overcooked. If the rice has been overcooked, you will find yourself trying to stir-fry a gummy mess. Trust me, it's like nailing Jell-O to the wall.

I store containers of cooked rice in my freezer (Ball makes amazing screw-top plastic containers that are freezer safe.) This way, I can have a quick dinner anytime with little planning other than defrosting the rice in the refrigerator, either overnight or during the workday.

4 tablespoons canola or other neutral oil, for stir-frying

3 extra-large eggs, lightly beaten

2 scallions, white and green parts chopped finely

4 cups cold, previously cooked rice, with the grains separated as
     much as possible

1 teaspoon toasted sesame oil

2 tablespoons gluten-free tamari, plus more to taste

1 teaspoon rice wine vinegar

1. Heat a wok or large skillet over high heat and add 2 tablespoons of the canola oil. When the oil is hot, add the eggs. Stir to scramble the eggs, and cook only until slightly runny. Remove the eggs from the pan and set them aside. Wipe out the pan.

2. Add the remaining 2 tablespoons of canola oil to the hot pan. Add the scallions and the rice, and stir, spreading the rice in a shallow layer in the pan. Allow to cook for about 2 minutes without stirring. Using a wooden spoon, break the rice apart, then stir in the sesame oil, tamari, and rice vinegar.

3. Return the cooked egg to the pan, and mix well. Serve immediately.

Baked Falafel

MAKES 4 SERVINGS

Time Estimate: 30 minutes active time,
15 minutes inactive time, including making pita

Can be doubled or halved easily

....

Soaking the dried chickpeas really does make all the difference in this recipe. So it generally does take a bit of planning. But if you don't want to plan ahead or if planning is simply not your strong suit as it generally isn't mine, just place the dried chickpeas with enough water to cover them by 2 inches in the pressure cooker, bring to pressure, and cook for 5 minutes on HIGH (15 dpi). Then drain and proceed with the recipe. But if all you have are canned chickpeas, make something else tonight or you'll be terribly disappointed in your falafel. One final note: The very same recipe can, of course, also be deep-fried in 350°F oil. But baking, rather than frying, makes for a lighter falafel, and a considerably quicker and less messy dinner.

1 cup dried chickpeas, soaked overnight covered with 2 inches water and then
    drained (or pressure cooker alternative; see headnote)

1 medium-size yellow onion, peeled and chopped roughly

5 cloves garlic, smashed and peeled

1 teaspoon kosher salt

¼ teaspoon Mexican chili powder, or to taste

2 teaspoons ground cumin

1 teaspoon baking powder

1 tablespoon sesame tahini (optional)

6 tablespoons (54 g) high-quality all-purpose gluten-free flour

¼ cup roughly chopped fresh parsley leaves

¼ cup roughly chopped fresh cilantro leaves

Extra-virgin olive oil, as needed

Yeast-Free Pita Bread, for serving (page 57)

Hummus, for serving

1. Preheat your oven to 400°F. Line a rimmed baking sheet with unbleached parchment paper and set it aside.

2. In the bowl of your food processor fitted with the steel blade, place the chick-peas and pulse them a few times until chopped but not pureed. Add the onion, garlic, salt, chili powder, cumin, baking powder, and the tahini (if using), and pulse until well blended. Add the flour, parsley, and cilantro, and pulse a few times until the mixture starts to clump together.

3. Turn on the food processor. Drizzle in olive oil very slowly only until the mixture begins to come together in a ball. Turn out the dough onto a lightly floured piece of unbleached parchment paper and press together.

4. With wet hands, divide the dough into twenty-four pieces and roll each tightly into a ball. Place about 1 inch apart on the prepared baking sheet, then drizzle each ball liberally with olive oil to ensure browning in the oven. Place the baking sheet in the freezer for about 10 minutes, or until the balls are firm.

5. If making pita bread, begin to make the dough.

6. Place the baking sheet with the falafel in the preheated oven and bake until lightly golden brown on the top and browned on the underside, about 15 minutes. Finish making the pita bread dough.

7. When the falafel is done baking, remove from the oven. Place the pita bread dough in the oven and bake according to the recipe directions. Serve the falafel in the pita, with hummus.

Shoestring Savings

On a shoestring: 72¢/serving

If you bought it: $2.10/serving (frozen)

Refrigerator Pizza Dough White Pizza

MAKES TWO 10-INCH PIZZAS

Time Estimate: 23 minutes active time, 12 minutes inactive time

Can be doubled or halved easily

Whenever I make white pizza, I have to restrain myself. I really just want to cover the whole top with ricotta cheese, because melted ricotta is one of life's greatest pleasures. I remind myself that too much is, indeed, called "too much" for a reason. It makes the pizza heavy with moisture, making it wilt.

1 recipe Yeasted Refrigerator Pizza Dough (page 63)

1 small yellow onion, peeled and diced

2 cloves garlic, smashed and peeled

2 tablespoons extra-virgin olive oil

8 ounces shredded mozzarella cheese

½ cup finely grated Parmigiano-Reggiano

6 ounces ricotta cheese (whole milk or part skim)

1. Preheat your oven to 425°F. Place a pizza stone (or an overturned rimmed baking sheet, if you don't have one) on the bottom rack of the oven as it heats.

2. Divide the pizza dough into two pieces. Place one piece on a lightly floured piece of unbleached parchment paper, dust the dough lightly with flour, cover with another sheet of unbleached parchment paper, and roll into an 12-inch round. Remove the top sheet of parchment paper. Roll in the edges to create a crust, and pinch to secure. Repeat with the second piece of dough.

3. Place each crust, one at a time, still on a piece of parchment paper, on the hot pizza stone or overturned baking sheet. Bake for about 5 minutes, or until the crust begins to stiffen a bit.

4. While the crusts are baking, in a medium-size skillet, sauté the onion and garlic in the olive oil over medium-high heat, stirring frequently, until the onion is translucent and the garlic is fragrant, about 6 minutes.

5. Once they are finished parbaking, remove the crusts from the oven. Divide the onion mixture between the two pizzas and spread over the pizza crust, up to

about an inch from the edge. Scatter the mozzarella and Parmigiano-Reggiano on top of each pizza. Scatter dollops of half of the ricotta cheese on one pizza, and the rest on the other pizza.

6. Bake the pizzas, one at a time, on the hot pizza stone or overturned baking sheet for about 7 minutes each, or until the cheese is melted and bubbling and the crust is beginning to brown. Allow the cheese to set for a couple of minutes before slicing and serving.

Vegetable Calzones

MAKES 4 SERVINGS

Time Estimate: 25 minutes active time, 15 minutes inactive time

Can be doubled or halved easily

....

As if I haven't said enough about how useful that Yeasted Refrigerator Pizza Dough (page 63) is, here's proof positive.

1 recipe Yeasted Refrigerator Pizza Dough (page 63)

2 to 3 tablespoons extra-virgin olive oil

1 small onion, peeled and diced

2 cloves garlic, peeled and minced

4 ounces pancetta, cubed (optional)

1 (8-ounce) package sliced button mushrooms

1 (1-pound) bag fresh triple-washed spinach

Kosher salt and freshly ground black pepper

15 to 16 ounces ricotta cheese (whole milk or part skim)

1 cup finely grated Parmigiano-Reggiano cheese

½ cup grated Gruyère or white Cheddar cheese

2 extra-large eggs, beaten

2 tablespoons chopped fresh basil, or 1 tablespoon dried

2 tablespoons chopped fresh oregano, or 1 tablespoon dried

1 tablespoon unsalted butter, melted, mixed with 1 tablespoon
    extra-virgin olive oil, for brushing

1. Preheat your oven to 425°F. Place a pizza stone (or an overturned rimmed baking sheet, if you don't have one) in the oven as it heats.

2. Divide the pizza dough into four equal portions and roll each into a ball. Set the dough aside, covered loosely with a wet towel.

3. In a medium-size saucepan, combine 2 tablespoons of the olive oil with the onion. Sauté, stirring frequently, over medium heat, until the onion is translucent, about 5 minutes. Add the minced garlic, pancetta (if using), and mushrooms, and sauté, stirring frequently, until the garlic is fragrant, the pancetta is cooked, and

the mushrooms have begun to soften, about 6 minutes. Transfer the mushroom mixture to a large bowl.

4. Add the fresh spinach to the saucepan and cook over high heat, stirring frequently, until wilted, about a minute, and add to the bowl containing the mushroom mixture. Mix well, adding salt and pepper to taste. If you haven't used the pancetta, you will need more salt. Set the bowl aside to cool.

5. Take the first ball of pizza dough and roll it out between two pieces of lightly floured unbleached parchment paper into a 6- to 8-inch round about ⅛ inch thick (thickness of a nickel). If the edges are very rough, tuck them toward the center of the round and then roll them smooth. Repeat with the remaining balls of dough.

6. To the large bowl, add the ricotta, grated cheeses, and eggs, and mix well. Fold in the basil and oregano.

7. Divide the filling among the four rounds of pizza dough, placing the filling on half of each round, leaving a 1-inch border of bare dough. Fold the opposite end of the dough over the filling and pinch together the edges well until there is a good seal. Brush the tops and seams with the butter mixture.

8. Place the calzones on unbleached parchment paper, and place the parchment paper on top of the pizza stone or overturned baking sheet. Bake until nicely browned and crisp, about 15 minutes. Serve immediately.

Shoestring Savings

On a shoestring: $4.16 each
If you bought it: $7.95 each

Yeast-Free Pizza Margherita

MAKES 2 10-INCH PIZZAS

Time Estimate: 20 minutes active time, 10 minutes inactive time

Can be doubled or halved easily

....

You were hoping to serve pizza for dinner tonight, but you come home and realize that you're all out of Yeasted Refrigerator Pizza Dough! What now? You can't very well throw in the towel and ask your family very sweetly if they wouldn't mind waiting until breakfast to eat. (I've tried. Doesn't work.) A quick dinner is still only 30 minutes away. Here's how.

1 recipe Yeast-Free Pizza Dough (page 65)

1 cup tomato sauce

½ cup chopped fresh basil

¼ cup chopped fresh parsley (optional)

½ cup finely grated Parmigiano-Reggiano

8 ounces fresh mozzarella cheese, sliced into ¼-inch thick rounds

1. Preheat your oven to 425°F. Grease a large cast-iron skillet or tart pan well with unsalted butter, and set it aside.

2. Roll out the pizza dough between two sheets of lightly floured unbleached parchment paper and carefully tuck it into the bottom and halfway up the sides of the prepared skillet or tart pan. If rolling it out makes the dough too difficult to handle, with wet hands, simply press it into the bottom of the skillet or pan and up the sides.

3. Spread the tomato sauce all over the bottom of the crust. Place the skillet in the hot oven for about 5 minutes, or until the crust begins to stiffen a bit. Remove the pan from the oven. *longer. bottom tasted a bit doughy*

4. Scatter the chopped basil and parsley, and then the grated cheese, on top of the sauce. Blot the rounds of mozzarella cheese with paper towels and scatter them over the top.

5. Place the skillet pizza in the hot oven, and bake for about 10 minutes, or until the cheese is melted and bubbling and the crust is beginning to brown. Allow the cheese to set for a couple minutes before slicing and serving.

VARIATIONS: Instead of sauce, herbs, and cheese on your yeast-free pizza, try making yeast-free Refrigerator Pizza Dough White Pizza (page 106) or Pesto Chicken Pizza (page 147) with or without the chicken.

Shoestring Savings

On a shoestring: $4.42/pizza

If you bought it: $8.93/pizza (frozen)

Vegetarian Chili

MAKES 4 SERVINGS

Time Estimate: 10 minutes active time, 15 minutes inactive time

Can be doubled or halved easily

....

This is a basic, quick veggie chili recipe. Hearty and satisfying, it's ready in a flash. To dial it up a bit, make Chili Pie. Cook the chili as directed, and then divide among four 6-inch ramekins. Top with squares of Basic Pastry Crust (page 85), brush the crust with milk, and bake at 375°F for 20 minutes, or until the crust is browned and the filling is bubbling.

1 small onion, peeled and diced

2 cloves garlic, peeled and minced

2 tablespoons extra-virgin olive oil

1 cup (8 ounces) prepared salsa

2 (15-ounce) cans black beans, drained and rinsed

1 (15-ounce) can red kidney beans, drained and rinsed

1 (28-ounce) can crushed tomatoes

¼ cup tomato paste

1 tablespoon ground cumin

1 teaspoon Mexican chili powder, or to taste

Kosher salt and freshly ground black peppe, to taste

2 cups vegetable stock

1. In a large, heavy-bottomed saucepan over medium heat, sauté the onion and garlic in the olive oil until the onion is translucent and the garlic is fragrant, about 6 minutes. Add the rest of the ingredients, and mix well.

2. With an immersion blender, puree about half the mixture. Turn the heat to medium-high and bring to a boil. Lower the heat to a simmer and allow to cook, uncovered, until reduced by about one-quarter, about 15 minutes. Serve immediately.

Shoestring Savings

On a shoestring: $2.06/serving

If you bought it: $3.20/serving

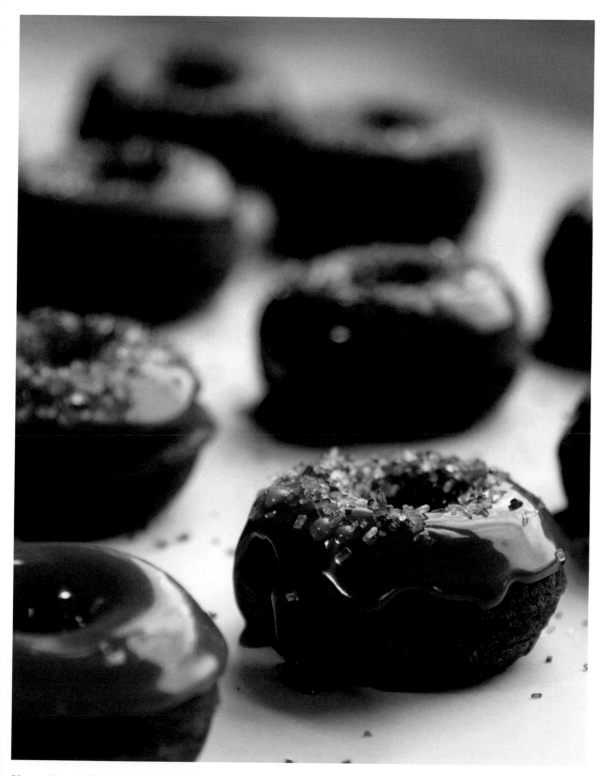

Yeast-Free Glazed Chocolate Doughnuts. PAGE 44.

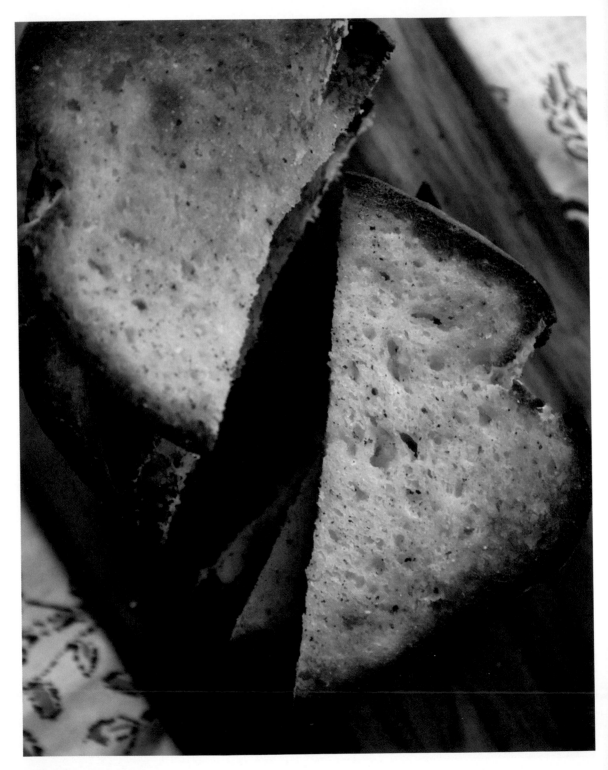

Texas Toast. PAGE 48.

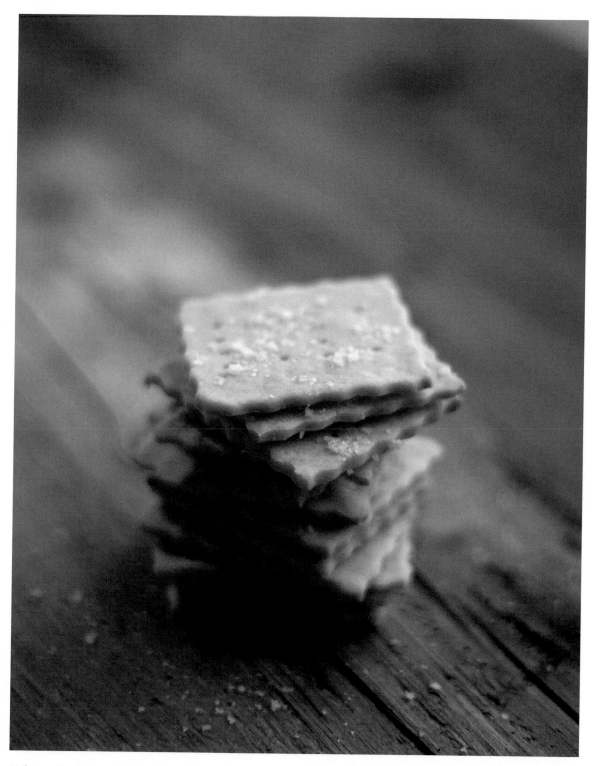

Saltine-Style Crackers. PAGE 74.

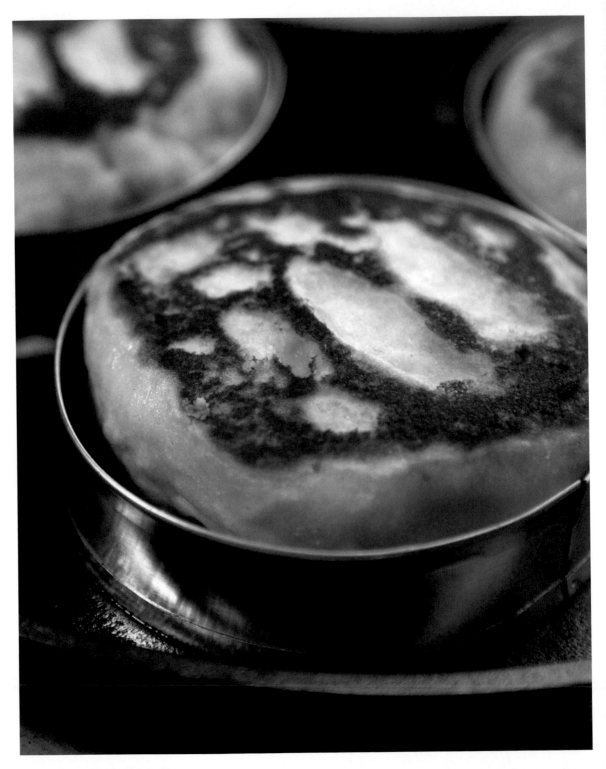

Yeast-Free English Muffins. PAGE 55.

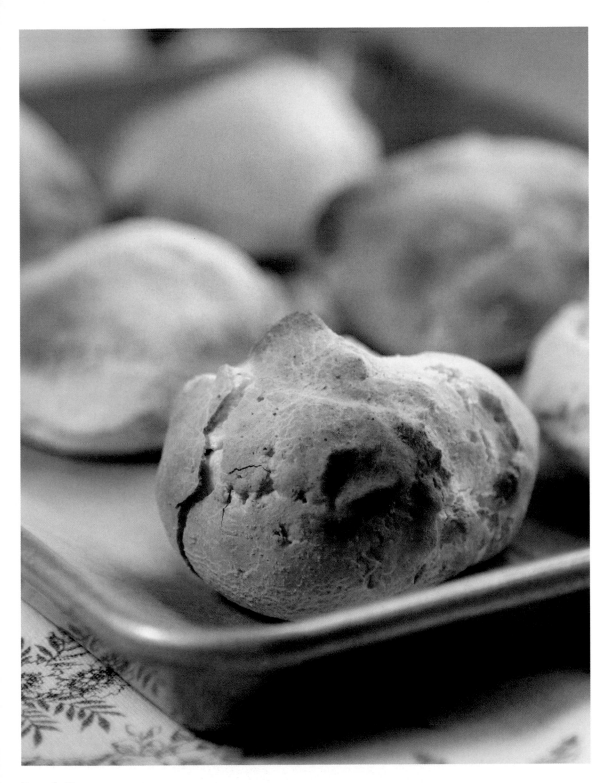

Pan de Bono. PAGE 78.

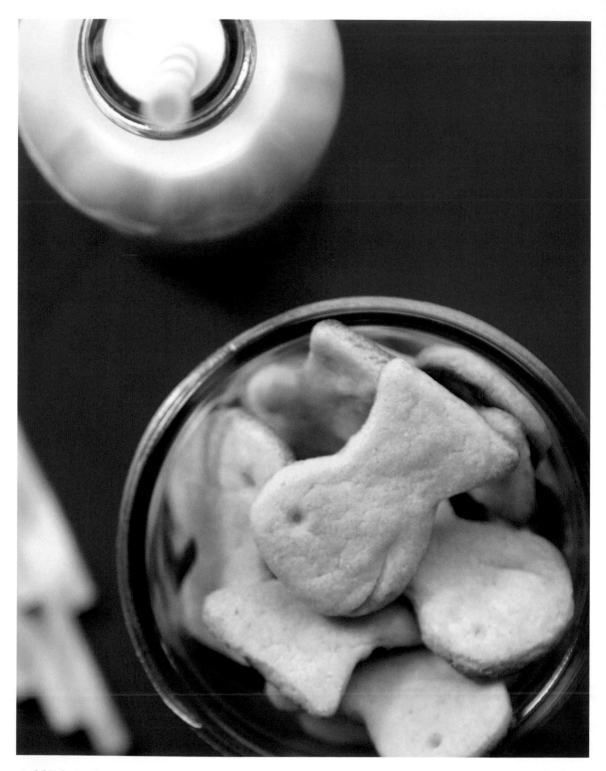

Goldfish-Style Crackers. PAGE 76.

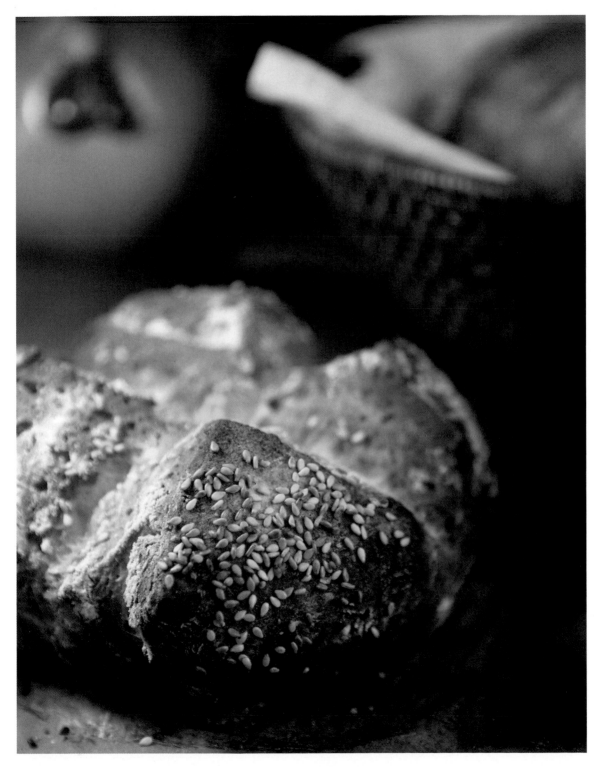

Boule Bread with Yeasted Refrigerator Bread Dough. PAGE 72.

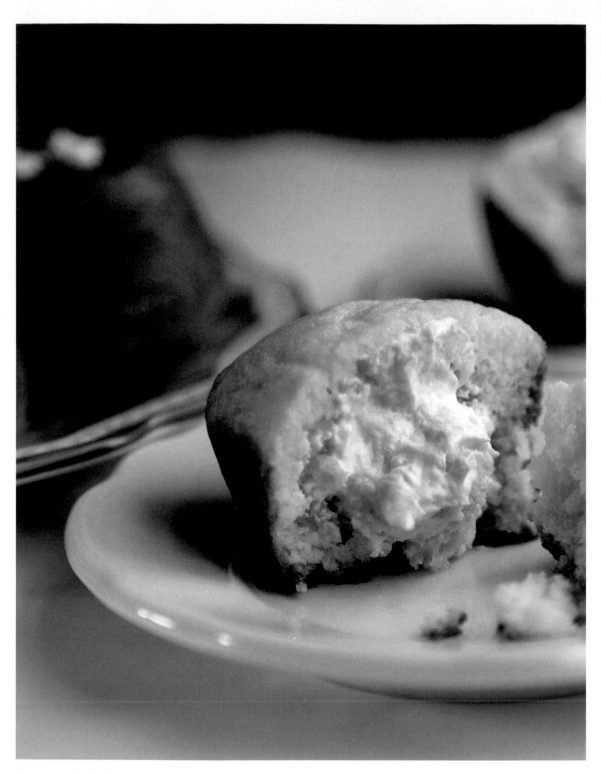

Twinkie-Style Cupcakes. PAGE 154.

Tomato and Corn Risotto

MAKES 4 SERVINGS

Time Estimate: 30 minutes active time, 10 minutes inactive time

Can be doubled or halved easily

Did you think that risotto was just too difficult or temperamental, or that it just took too long for a weeknight? Pish posh. Risotto is another meal with so many possible variations, it's a wonder it doesn't show up on everyone's dinner table at least once a week. Follow the directions precisely and you'll soon get a feel for how you can shake it up by replacing the tomatoes and corn with whatever is in season. And be sure not to cook with any wine you wouldn't drink. Cooking it down intensifies its flavor.

1 medium-size yellow onion, peeled and diced

4 tablespoons (56 g) unsalted butter

2 cups uncooked Arborio rice

½ cup dry white wine (e.g., Pinot Grigio)

3½ to 4 cups good vegetable stock

Kosher salt and freshly ground black pepper, to taste

1 dry pint (2 cups) grape tomatoes, halved

Cooked corn from 2 ears

1. In a large, enameled cast-iron Dutch oven or nonstick stockpot, sauté the onion in the butter over medium-high heat, stirring occasionally, until the onion is translucent, about 6 minutes.

2. Add the rice and cook, stirring frequently, until the rice has become somewhat translucent, about 2 minutes. Add the white wine, stir, and continue to cook, stirring occasionally, until the alcohol evaporates, about 2 minutes.

3. Add 2½ cups of vegetable stock, stir, lower the heat to medium, and continue to cook, stirring occasionally, until the liquid is mostly absorbed, about 10 minutes.

4. Add at least another cup of stock by the ladleful, stirring frequently, until the liquid is mostly absorbed. Continue to add stock until the rice is al dente (you'll have to taste-test to determine) and the risotto is creamy. Add salt and pepper to taste.

5. Remove the risotto from the heat, stir in the tomatoes and corn, and serve immediately.

Chapter 6
....

Weekday Workday Dinners

The way I handle a week's worth of dinners is by compartmentalizing. It goes something like this.

Friday nights are pizza nights, and I always have Yeasted Refrigerator Pizza Dough (page 63) on hand. Done, and now we're down to four weeknights.

If I have a loose idea of what I'd like to make on three of those four nights, I can use that to inform my grocery shopping for the week. So at least I have the fresh meats and vegetables I need to make some weeknight magic happen. I figure on one night for a beef-based meal such as *albondigas*, one night for a chicken dish such as a pressure cooker chicken soup or quick chicken fajitas. Only two nights unaccounted for. One can be a vegetarian meal from Chapter 5, and the other, I figure I'll fly by the seat of my pants. I can handle one night that's a wild card. No biggie.

- One-Pot Albondigas Dinner
- Pancetta Meatball Soup
- One-Pot Baked Sole and Soppressata Dinner
- One-Pot Sausage Meatballs Dinner
- Chicken Meatballs
- Speedy Chicken Enchiladas
- Weeknight Chicken Soup

- Chicken Fajitas
- Quick Chicken Pot Pie
- Quick Shepherd's Pie
- Skillet Chicken and Tomatoes
- White Bean, Spinach, and Tomato Stew with Cheese Toast
- Chicken Quesadillas
- Masa-Stuffed Chicken
- Beef and Cheese Burritos
- Beef Taquitos
- Pesto Chicken Pizza

One-Pot Albondigas Dinner

MAKES 4 TO 6 SERVINGS

Time Estimate: 15 minutes active time, 25 minutes inactive time

Can be doubled or halved easily

···

Want to make this even speedier? Mix and shape the raw meatballs up to a day ahead of time. Omit the onion and garlic and just use good, really flavorful tomato sauce with lots of onions and garlic. Omit the pasta if you like to serve as a thinner soup, and you'll shave almost 10 minutes off your cooking time. This makes a large amount of food, and the leftovers taste even better the next day.

1 large onion, peeled and diced

4 tablespoons extra-virgin olive oil

1 large clove garlic, peeled and minced

4 cups chicken or vegetable stock

5½ cups water

1 cup tomato sauce

2 extra-large eggs plus one extra-large egg yolk, lightly beaten

⅔ cup uncooked short-grain white rice (such as Arborio)

2 pounds lean ground beef

Handful of fresh mint leaves, chopped finely

Handful of fresh parsley, chopped finely

2 teaspoons dried oregano, or a handful of fresh, chopped

1 teaspoon kosher salt

¼ teaspoon freshly ground black pepper

½ pound dried, short gluten-free pasta

1. In a 6- to 7-quart heavy-bottomed stockpot, sauté the onion in the olive oil over medium heat until translucent, about 6 minutes, stirring occasionally. Add the garlic and cook until fragrant, about 2 minutes more. Turn the heat to medium-high and add the stock, water, and tomato sauce. Cover the pot and bring to a boil, then lower the heat to a simmer.

2. While the liquid is simmering, place the eggs and rice in a large bowl and mix well. Add the ground beef, mint, parsley, oregano, salt, and pepper, and mix gently to combine.

3. Form meatballs about 1½ inches in diameter. Do not pack them too tightly or they will take too long to cook. Carefully add the meatballs to the pot of simmering liquid. Cover and let cook for 20 to 25 minutes, or until the meatballs are cooked through.

4. Remove the meatballs from the liquid with a strainer and set them aside. Add the dried pasta to the simmering soup and cook according to the package directions, stirring occasionally, until al dente.

5. Ladle the liquid and pasta to serve, and top with cooked meatballs.

Pancetta Meatball Soup

MAKES 4 TO 5 SERVINGS
Time Estimate: 15 minutes active time, 25 minutes inactive time
Can be doubled or halved easily

....

I buy vacuum-packed, 4-ounce packages of pancetta, already cubed. It's sold for a surprisingly reasonable price, and it is the understated highlight of any meal in which it appears. It certainly helps make quick work of this meatball soup.

4 cups beef or vegetable stock

2 cups water

1½ cups tomato sauce

4 extra-large egg yolks

½ teaspoon kosher salt

¼ teaspoon freshly ground black pepper

Leaves from 4 sprigs of fresh thyme, or ¾ teaspoon dried

1 pound lean ground beef

4 ounces cubed pancetta

2 ounces Parmigiano-Reggiano, grated finely

1. In a large Dutch oven or stockpot over medium-high heat, bring the stock, water, and tomato sauce to a boil.

2. While the liquid comes to a boil, in a large bowl, place the egg yolks, salt, pepper, and thyme, and whisk with a fork to mix well. Add the ground beef, pancetta, and grated cheese, and mix well with a large spoon or your hands. Divide the meat mixture into thirty portions. With wet hands, roll each into a ball. Do not roll the meatballs too tightly, or they will cook too slowly.

3. One by one, carefully add the meatballs to the boiling stock. Return to a boil, then lower the heat to medium. Cover the pot and allow to simmer for about 25 minutes, or until the meatballs are cooked through, removing the lid for the final 5 minutes to allow the liquid to reduce a bit. Serve the soup hot, with a slice of crusty gluten-free bread.

One-Pot Baked Sole and Soppressata Dinner

MAKES 4 SERVINGS

Time Estimate: 15 minutes active time, 15 minutes inactive time

Can be doubled or halved easily

....

Fish is not something I make too often at home, as it tends to be expensive. But if you are better at planning than I am, ask the fishmonger at your local market to recommend a brand of frozen fish. Then follow the package directions for thawing the fish on the day you plan to serve it for dinner. And if you have a Trader Joe's nearby, its frozen fish selection is a thing to behold. Remember that, unless you live in a fishing village, the fish you buy unfrozen has already been frozen and then thawed, just as you might do yourself at home.

4 tablespoons extra-virgin olive oil

2 tablespoons (28 g) unsalted butter

½ cup peeled and chopped shallots

4 ounces soppressata, thinly sliced

1 pound red skin potatoes, washed and sliced ¼ inch thick

1½ cups chicken or vegetable stock

¼ teaspoon saffron threads (optional)

Kosher salt and freshly ground black pepper, to taste

1 (1-pound) bag triple-washed fresh baby spinach (optional)

1½ pounds fillet of sole

1. Preheat your oven to 425°F. Heat 3 tablespoons of the oil plus the butter over medium-high heat in a large Dutch oven or heavy-bottomed, oven-safe skillet. Add the chopped shallots and cook, stirring frequently, until mostly translucent, about 4 minutes.

2. Add the sliced *soppressata* and cook over medium-high heat until softened and beginning to brown, about 2 minutes.

3. Add the potatoes, stock, saffron (if using), salt, and pepper, and stir. Bring to a boil and cook, mostly covered, for about 5 minutes to allow the potatoes to

begin to soften. Add the spinach leaves (if using) and cover once more to wilt the spinach, about 1 minute.

4. Season the sole with salt and pepper, remove the cover from the pot, and place the fish on top of the potato mixture. Drizzle the remaining tablespoon of olive oil over the fish. Cook, uncovered, until the sole is opaque throughout, 5 to 7 minutes. Serve immediately with a piece of crusty gluten-free bread.

One-Pot Sausage Meatballs Dinner

MAKES 4 TO 6 SERVINGS
Time Estimate: 15 minutes active time, 30 minutes inactive time
Can be doubled or halved easily

If you're ever lucky enough to find bulk sweet Italian sausage (no casings) for sale, buy it and make it that night! I can't seem to figure out whether it tastes better because there's less work for me, or whether they put a little something extra in there when they sell it in bulk. Try it as described in this sausage meatball recipe, or just brown it, mix it with some good tomato sauce, and serve it over al dente pasta. Just don't forget to ask the butcher about their safe food-handling practices to be sure your sausage is free from cross-contamination—and that it has no gluten-containing filler.

4 cups beef or vegetable stock

2 cups water

Kosher salt and freshly ground black pepper, to taste

5 extra-large egg yolks

1 teaspoon smoked Spanish paprika

1 pound lean ground beef

1 pound gluten-free sweet Italian sausage, casings removed

1½ cups tomato sauce

1 pound dried, short gluten-free pasta

1. In a large, enameled cast-iron Dutch oven or stockpot over medium-high heat, bring the stock and water to a boil. Season to taste with salt and pepper.

2. While the liquid is coming to a boil, place the egg yolks and paprika in a large bowl and whisk with a fork to mix well. Add the ground beef and sausage, and mix gently but well with a large spoon or your hands. Divide the meat into eighteen portions. With wet hands, roll each into a ball. Be careful not to pack the meatballs too tightly or they will cook too slowly.

3. Once the liquid is boiling, one by one, carefully add the meatballs. Return to a boil, then lower the heat to medium.

4. Cover the pot and allow to simmer for 20 to 30 minutes, or until the meatballs are cooked through. Transfer the meatballs to a platter and set them aside. Add the tomato sauce and then the pasta to the hot liquid and cook, stirring occasionally, until cooked to the desired consistency, according to the package directions.

5. Serve the meatballs over the pasta.

Chicken Meatballs

MAKES 4 SERVINGS

Time Estimate: 15 minutes active time, 20 minutes inactive time

Can be doubled or halved easily

....

My family loves meat loaf, but I love meatballs of all kinds even better. They come together just as quickly, they're easy to pack with flavor, and they cook so much faster than a large meat loaf does. These chicken meatballs are a nice change of pace from traditional meatballs, and can help make chicken an easier sell if you have any pint-size family members who are currently boycotting chicken—as each of my three children did at one point or another.

1½ pounds ground chicken (or an equal amount skinless boneless chicken
     breasts, diced)

2 extra-large eggs, at room temperature, lightly beaten

8 ounces cream cheese, at room temperature

10 ounces frozen whole-leaf spinach, thawed and squeezed dry

2 ounces Parmigiano-Reggiano, grated finely

¾ cup gluten-free bread crumbs

3 cloves garlic, peeled and minced

Leaves from 3 sprigs fresh thyme, or ¾ teaspoon dried

1 tablespoon extra-virgin olive oil

1 tablespoon (14 g) unsalted butter, melted and cooled

1 teaspoon kosher salt

¼ teaspoon freshly ground black pepper

    1. Preheat your oven to 400°F. Line a rimmed baking sheet with nonstick (or greased) aluminum foil.

    2. In a large bowl, place all of the ingredients and mix well.

3. Form the mixture into twenty meatballs, each about 1 inch in diameter, using a spring-loaded ice-cream scoop. Place the meatballs about 1 inch apart on the prepared pan, and shape into proper balls, using wet hands, if necessary.

4. Bake in the center of the oven for about 20 minutes, or until the meatballs are firm and an instant-read thermometer inserted into the center reads 165°F. Serve over pasta or rice.

Speedy Chicken Enchiladas

MAKES 6 SERVINGS

Time Estimate: 15 minutes active time, 15 minutes inactive time

Can be doubled or halved easily

....

I love to make my own enchilada sauce, all smoky with one of my favorite spices, smoked Spanish paprika. But there are actually some really nice prepared enchilada sauces that are gluten-free and really flavorful, for when you just don't have the time or the inclination. So far, my favorite is Hatch 5-Pepper Enchilada Sauce. I buy it mild, because I'm a bit of a wimp, but I'm sure you're much brawnier than me. Cubed rotisserie chicken helps this dish come together in a snap.

1 small yellow onion, peeled and diced

4 tablespoons extra-virgin olive oil

1 can (about 4.5 ounces) chopped green chiles, or 1 small jalapeño pepper, seeds and ribs removed, chopped

Kosher salt and freshly ground black pepper, to taste

2 cups cubed gluten-free rotisserie chicken

Juice of 1 lemon

1 (1-pound) bag triple-washed fresh baby spinach

1 recipe Flour Tortillas (page 80), or 8 to 10 gluten-free corn tortillas

2 cups sour cream or crème fraîche

1½ to 2 cups good, store-bought gluten-free enchilada sauce (such as Hatch 5-Pepper Enchilada Sauce)

2 ½ cups mixed shredded Monterey Jack and Cheddar cheeses

1. Preheat your oven to 400°F.

2. In a medium-size saucepan over medium heat, sauté the diced onion in the oil until translucent, about 6 minutes. Add the chopped green chiles. If using fresh, sauté over medium heat until softened, about 3 minutes more. If using canned, remove the pan from the heat and stir just to mix. Add salt and pepper to taste.

3. Transfer the onion mixture to a medium-size bowl. Add the cubed chicken and lemon juice to the bowl, and stir gently.

4. In the same medium-size saucepan, add the spinach and a splash of water to the pan, then cover and cook the spinach over medium heat until wilted, about a minute or two. Add the wilted spinach to the chicken mixture and stir gently.

5. Warm the tortillas in the microwave on HIGH for about 30 seconds, wrapped in wet paper towels. Lay out the warm tortillas on your work surface, and divide the chicken and spinach filling evenly among them, placing the mixture just off-center on top of each tortilla. Layer with sour cream or crème fraîche and a drizzling of enchilada sauce. Divide 1½ cups of the cheese among the tortillas, placing the cheese on top of the drizzled sauce.

6. Gently roll the tortillas to enclose the filling and place them, touching side to side and seam side down, in a 9 by 13-inch baking dish.

7. Cover the tortillas evenly with the remaining enchilada sauce, and then with the remaining shredded cheese. Bake in the center of the oven until the cheese is melted and the sauce is bubbling, about 10 minutes. Serve immediately.

Shoestring Savings

On a shoestring: $2.77/serving

If you bought it: $3.84/serving (frozen)

Weeknight Chicken Soup

MAKES 4 TO 6 SERVINGS

Time Estimate: 20 minutes active time, 20 minutes inactive time

Can be doubled or halved easily

....

Chicken soup with rice is medicine for whatever ails you. Be it a bad day or a bad cold, this dish has the power to make everything better. It used to be something I only cooked up on weekends, until I discovered how fast it is to make in a pressure cooker. If you've never used a modern pressure cooker before, they're safe nowadays. And they're a dream come true for those of us who want slow-cooked flavor in a flash. On a weeknight. When you're tired. And maybe in need of some tender loving care.

2 pounds skin-on, bone-in chicken thighs

1 large yellow onion, peeled and quartered

2 cloves garlic, peeled and smashed

2 large carrots, peeled and chopped

2 stalks celery, cleaned and chopped

2 dried bay leaves

2 cups chicken or vegetable stock

2 large sweet potatoes, peeled and diced

2 sprigs fresh thyme, or 1 teaspoon dried

Kosher salt and freshly ground black pepper, to taste

3 cups cooked brown or white rice

1. Place all the ingredients, except the rice, in a pressure cooker that has at least a 6-quart capacity, preferably 8-quart. Add enough cold water from the tap to bring the level to just below your pressure cooker's fill line.

2. Close and lock the lid of the pressure cooker securely and bring the pot to pressure over medium-high heat. Lower the heat to medium and cook for 16 minutes on HIGH (15 psi) or 28 minutes on LOW (8 psi) pressure.

3. Once the cooking time has ended, remove the pressure cooker from the heat and allow the pressure to drop naturally. Once the pressure has fallen enough for

the pressure indicator to lower, carefully remove the cover. Skim any impurities from the top of the liquid and remove and discard the two bay leaves and the two bare sprigs of thyme.

4. Remove the chicken thighs from the liquid. Skin and debone the chicken, which should fall away easily from the bone. If desired, puree the remaining soup ingredients with an immersion blender.

5. Shred the chicken meat and return it to the liquid. Add the cooked rice, and serve immediately.

Shoestring Savings

On a shoestring: $1.18/serving

If you bought it: $4.59/serving (frozen)

Chicken Fajitas

MAKES 4 SERVINGS

Time Estimate: 20 minutes active time, 10 minutes inactive time

Can be doubled or halved easily

I always marinate raw chicken in a gallon-size resealable plastic bag. Not only does it allow me to make sure that marinade covers every piece of chicken, but it makes cleanup a breeze (and safer, too, because of the dangers of handling raw meat). Here's another tip: Cut the chicken into strips before you marinate it. It will soak up a lot of the marinade, and the chicken will cook through more quickly. To save even more time on a weeknight, marinate the chicken the night before or in the morning before you start your day. When you're ready for dinner, it's almost ready for you.

2 pounds skinless, boneless chicken breast, cut into strips

Juice of 1 lemon

Juice of 2 limes

2 tablespoons neutral oil, such as canola

½ teaspoon kosher salt, or to taste

¼ teaspoon freshly ground black pepper, or to taste

1 large onion, peeled and quartered

3 cloves garlic, smashed and peeled

1 red bell pepper, seeded and roughly chopped

½ pound (about 3 medium-size round) tomatoes, chopped roughly

½ teaspoon ground cumin

½ teaspoon smoked Spanish paprika

Dash (⅛ teaspoon) of Mexican chili powder

½ teaspoon dried oregano

¼ teaspoon ground cinnamon

2 teaspoons sugar

8 gluten-free corn tortillas, or 6 Flour Tortillas (page 80), warmed

1. Place the raw chicken in a gallon-size resealable plastic bag, followed by the lemon and lime juices. Seal the bag and allow the chicken to marinate while you make the sauce.

2. In a large, heavy-bottomed saucepan, place the oil, salt, and pepper, and set the pan aside.

3. Place the onion, garlic, red pepper, tomatoes, cumin, paprika, chili powder, oregano, cinnamon, and sugar in a blender. Pulse until coarsely blended. Pour the blend into the large saucepan and sauté over medium-high heat, stirring frequently, until the onion is translucent and the garlic is fragrant, about 5 minutes.

4. Add the marinated chicken strips to the pan and lower the heat to medium-low. Cook, stirring occasionally, until the chicken is opaque and cooked through, about 10 minutes. Serve immediately with warmed tortillas.

Quick Chicken Pot Pie

MAKES 4 SERVINGS (1 LARGE POTPIE)
Time Estimate: 20 minutes active time, 20 minutes inactive time
Can be doubled or halved easily

....

The slower version of this recipe starts with a roux (a cooked mixture of equal parts fat, such as clarified butter, and flour) to thicken the pie filling. Here, I jumped ahead by adding some mascarpone cheese. This recipe also calls for skinless, boneless chicken breast that cooks right in the pot, and it makes one large pot pie rather than individual pies for each person. Sometimes a few tweaks are all it takes to shortcut a slow-cooked favorite without sacrificing flavor. And if you keep some Basic Pastry Crust (page 85) on hand these days, this dish is possible even on a weeknight.

1 recipe Basic Pastry Crust, chilled (page 85)

4 tablespoons unsalted butter

4 tablespoons extra-virgin olive oil

3 medium-size carrots, peeled and chopped roughly

3 stalks celery, trimmed and chopped roughly

1 bunch scallions, trimmed, green and white parts chopped

Kosher salt and freshly ground black pepper

2 cups chicken stock

2 pounds skinless, boneless chicken breast, cut into bite-size pieces

1 tablespoon spicy mustard

8 ounces mascarpone cheese

Leaves of 5 to 6 sprigs fresh thyme, or 1 to 1½ teaspoons dried thyme

Milk, for brushing

1. Roll out the pastry crust between two sheets of unbleached parchment paper into a 10-inch square (or about 2 inches larger than the width of the pan you intend to use). Return the crust to the refrigerator to chill, wrapped in its parchment paper.

2. Preheat your oven to 400°F. Grease a deep, 9-inch square baking pan and set it aside.

3. In a large, heavy-bottomed saucepan, place 2 tablespoons each of the butter and olive oil, along with the carrots, celery, and scallions, adding salt and pepper to taste. Cook over medium-high heat, stirring frequently, until the vegetables are glistening, about 8 minutes. Add the chicken stock, cover, and bring to a boil over medium-high heat. Lower the heat to a simmer and allow to cook uncovered.

4. While the vegetables simmer, cook the chicken. In a separate, medium-size pan, place the remaining 2 tablespoons each of the butter and olive oil, along with the chicken, salt, and pepper. Cook over medium-high heat until opaque throughout, about 3 minutes per side. Add the mustard, mascarpone cheese, and thyme, and stir.

5. Transfer the chicken mixture to the large pan of vegetables. Stir until well mixed. Ladle the entire mixture into the prepared baking dish.

6. Remove the crust from the refrigerator, peel back the parchment paper, and nestle the crust on top of the filling, tucking it over itself and pressing it down. With a sharp knife, slash the crust in a few places to prevent it from bubbling over. Brush the crust generously with milk.

7. Bake the pot pie in the center of the oven until golden brown and bubbling, about 15 minutes.

Quick Shepherd's Pie

MAKES 4 SERVINGS

Time Estimate: 15 minutes active time, 15 minutes inactive time

Can be doubled or halved easily

....

To some, using potato flakes or bits is second nature. To others, it feels like cheating. Wherever you fall on this contentious potato flakes continuum, try baking them. When you bake them on top of this quick shepherd's pie filling, they not only brown and get crispy on the edges, but they soak up all of that satisfying liquid below. And Idaho Spuds Brand Signature Potato Bits are truly superior to other brands. I order them on Amazon.com, but they might just be in a mainstream market near you.

1 pound extra-lean ground beef

⅓ cup tomato paste

2 tablespoons mascarpone cheese

2 teaspoons Worcestershire sauce

8 ounces frozen mixed vegetables, thawed and drained

2 cups Idaho Spuds Brand Signature Potato Bits, with the amounts water, milk,
    butter, and salt specified in package directions

4 ounces Cheddar cheese, shredded

Handful of fresh parsley leaves (optional), chopped roughly

1. Preheat your oven to 375°F. Grease a 9-inch square baking dish and set it aside.

2. Cook the beef in a large skillet over medium-high heat until browned throughout, 4 to 5 minutes.

3. Stir in the tomato paste, mascarpone cheese, and Worcestershire sauce. Add the mixed vegetables and stir until well mixed. Heat until the vegetables are warmed. Spoon the mixture into the prepared dish.

4. Prepare the mashed potatoes according to the package directions.

5. In a separate bowl, mix the shredded cheese with the potatoes, and gently stir in the chopped parsley (if using). Spread the mashed potato mixture evenly over the beef mixture.

6. Bake in the center of the oven until the potatoes are nicely browned on top, about 10 minutes. Serve immediately.

Skillet Chicken and Tomatoes

MAKES 4 SERVINGS

Time Estimate: 15 minutes active time, 10 minutes inactive time

Can be doubled or halved easily

....

This is a weeknight no-brainer, especially if you buy boneless chicken and tomatoes every week like I do. And I always have some dry white wine around, in case my chicken—or I—need some. Or you can use vermouth, which tends to be well priced and it can last a few days in the refrigerator once it's been opened.

4 tablespoons extra-virgin olive oil

1 tablespoon unsalted butter

1½ pounds skinless, boneless chicken breasts

Kosher salt and freshly ground black pepper, to taste

2 large cloves garlic, smashed and peeled

1 large lemon, washed

1 cup chicken stock

½ cup dry white wine (such as Pinot Grigio), or vermouth

1 dry pint (2 cups) grape tomatoes, halved

1. In a large, cast-iron skillet over medium-high heat, heat the oil and butter. Add as many of the chicken breasts as will fit without overlapping. Season with salt and pepper to taste. Add the crushed garlic to the hot pan. Slice the lemon into four wedges and scatter the pieces in the pan.

2. Add the stock and wine, and bring to a simmer (you will smell the alcohol burning off). Turn down the heat to medium and cook the chicken for about 4 minutes per side, until cooked all the way through. Remove the cooked chicken, add any uncooked pieces, and cook for 4 minutes per side.

3. Remove the chicken and lemon wedges from the pan, leaving behind the garlic. Add the tomatoes to the hot pan, and cook over medium-high heat until they just begin to soften, about 2 minutes. Simmer until the liquid is reduced by about one-fourth, about 7 minutes. Remove and discard the garlic.

4. Return the chicken to the pan and cook for a minute until warmed through. Serve the chicken and tomatoes immediately over cooked rice or quinoa.

White Bean, Spinach, and Tomato Stew with Cheese Toast

MAKES 4 SERVINGS

Time Estimate: 20 minutes active time, 10 minutes inactive time

Can be doubled or halved easily

....

This stew has that all-day cooked flavor without your having to cook all day. The secret? Shallots add lots of depth and flavor to the finished dish. And they are mild enough that even those who tend to object to onions don't mind or even necessarily detect their presence. I suggest serving this with cheese toast made with a Schär Parbaked Baguette, but any sort of bread will do. Because this dish cooks on the stovetop entirely, you can finish baking the bread in the toaster oven, rather than turning on the oven, for an even quicker meal.

4 medium-size shallots, peeled and chopped

5 tablespoons extra-virgin olive oil

3 cloves garlic, peeled and sliced very thinly

1 (1-pound) bag triple-washed fresh baby spinach

1 (28-ounce) can whole peeled tomatoes, chopped roughly

1 (15-ounce) can cannellini (white kidney) beans, drained and rinsed

2 generous tablespoons crème fraîche, softened cream cheese, or sour cream

1 cup vegetable or chicken stock

Leaves of 3 sprigs of fresh thyme or rosemary, or ¾ teaspoon dried

Kosher salt and freshly ground black pepper, to taste

1 gluten-free Schär Parbaked Baguette

½ pound fresh mozzarella cheese, sliced

1. In a large, cast-iron skillet over medium-high heat, cook the shallots in the oil until they soften, stirring frequently, about 3 minutes. Add the garlic and cook until fragrant, about another 2 minutes. Add the spinach, cover, and cook until wilted, about 1 minute. Add the tomatoes, beans, and cream, and stir. Add the stock, season to taste with the thyme, salt, and pepper, and stir to combine.

2. Cook uncovered over medium heat until the liquid is reduced a bit and the stew begins to thicken, about 7 minutes.

3. While the stew is reducing, slice the parbaked baguette into 1-inch-thick rounds. Toast both sides of the rounds in your toaster oven. Top with slices of mozzarella cheese and return the bread to the toaster oven for another few moments, until the cheese melts.

4. Serve the stew in large bowls, topped with a slice of cheese toast.

Chicken Quesadillas

MAKES 4 SERVINGS

Time Estimate: 20 minutes active time, 5 minutes inactive time

Can be doubled or halved easily

Most stores (even bulk goods stores such as Sam's Club and Costco) had been selling fully cooked, naturally gluten-free rotisserie chickens for ages before I had heard of such convenience. There I was, not realizing how a 10-minute car ride could save me hours of oven time. These days, it's open season on fully cooked birds at my house. I still buy raw chicken, of course, more often than not. But knowing that I have one of these fully cooked chickens sitting in my refrigerator, waiting to be transformed into chicken quesadillas in 25 minutes or less, helps me sleep just a little better at night.

1 small yellow onion, peeled and chopped

2 tablespoons neutral oil, like canola

1½ teaspoons ground cumin

¼ teaspoon Mexican chili powder

½ teaspoon kosher salt

½ cup vegetable or chicken stock

1 cup prepared salsa

2 to 3 cups shredded, cooked gluten-free rotisserie chicken

12 to 14 gluten-free corn tortillas

8 ounces sharp Cheddar cheese, or cheese of choice, shredded

1. Preheat your oven to 375°F. Line rimmed baking sheets with unbleached parchment paper and set them aside.

2. In a large, enameled cast-iron pot, sauté the onion in the oil over medium heat until the onion is translucent (about 6 minutes). Add the cumin, chili powder, and salt, and stir. Add the stock and salsa, and cook over medium-high heat, stirring occasionally, until the liquid from the stock and the salsa has begun to evaporate, 8 to 10 minutes. Turn off the heat and add the chicken, and allow the mixture to stand, uncovered.

3. Place the tortillas, one by one, in a dry, nonstick or cast-iron skillet over medium-low heat and cook both sides of each tortilla until it has begun to soften, about 30 seconds total per tortilla.

4. Place half of the tortillas on the prepared baking sheets. Divide the chicken mixture among the tortillas, placing it in the center of each tortilla and leaving at least a ½-inch border. Sprinkle generously with shredded cheese and top with the remaining tortillas.

5. Bake the quesadillas in the center of the oven until the cheese is melted and everything is warmed through, about 5 minutes. Slice in half or into wedges, and serve with sour cream and sliced or mashed avocado.

Masa-Stuffed Chicken

MAKES 4 SERVINGS

Time Estimate: 15 minutes active time, 20 minutes inactive time

Can be doubled or halved easily

Have I ever told you how much I love the precooked cornmeal called masa harina? I love it, not only for how deeply satisfying it tastes, but for how it looks and behaves, too. When you wet it with just enough water, it forms a gorgeous, smooth dough that won't stick to your hands. Because it is so easy to handle, especially once you gain some experience working with it, it makes for a very quick and hearty meal. When making this recipe, just be sure to create a pocket in each chicken breast that's deep enough to keep the filling from spilling right out while the chicken bakes.

2 pounds skinless, boneless chicken breast

1 small yellow onion, peeled and diced

2 tablespoons extra-virgin olive oil, plus more for drizzling

Garlic salt, to taste

Freshly ground black pepper, to taste

1 tablespoon dried oregano

1 (1-pound) bag triple-washed fresh baby spinach

⅓ cup (39 g) gluten-free masa harina (golden corn flour)

8 ounces Manchego (or other hard) cheese, shredded

¼ cup finely grated Parmigiano-Reggiano

1. Preheat your oven to 375°F. Line a rimmed baking sheet with nonstick or greased aluminum foil or unbleached parchment paper.

2. Slice each chicken breast horizontally into the center, without cutting all the way through, to create a pocket. Place the chicken breasts about 1 inch apart on the prepared baking sheet. Set aside.

3. In a medium-size skillet, cook the onion in 2 tablespoons of the olive oil over medium-high heat, stirring frequently, until the onion is translucent, about 6 minutes. Season with garlic salt and pepper. Rub the dried oregano in the palm

141

of one hand to release the oils, add it to the skillet, and stir. Add the spinach, toss to coat with the oil, and cover the pan. Allow the spinach to cook until it wilts, which will take just a minute. Remove the pan from the heat and scrape its contents into a medium-size, heat-safe bowl.

4. Add the masa harina to the bowl and stir well. Add the cheeses and stir well once again.

5. Scoop about 2 tablespoons of filling and stuff into the pocket of each chicken breast, with some filling peeking out of the pockets, and place the stuffed chicken on the prepared baking sheet. Drizzle the breasts with olive oil, and rub it in to all exposed areas of the meat. Season the chicken breasts with more garlic salt and pepper.

6. Bake in the center of the oven until the chicken is opaque throughout, about 20 minutes (depending upon the thickness of the breasts). Serve immediately.

Beef and Cheese Burritos

MAKES 4 TO 6 SERVINGS

Time Estimate: 25 minutes active time, 5 minutes inactive time

Can be doubled or halved easily

··

Making flour tortillas is a skill, like any other. You will get better and faster and just plain better (and faster) over time. Start off by making them on a day you have a bit of a time cushion, and you'll be amazed how quickly you can turn some flour and some ground beef and cheese into a complete burrito meal. And since burritos freeze beautifully, too, the batch you make on the weekend to perfect your technique? They can be dinner on Thursday night. Just thaw them in the refrigerator during the day and microwave for about 45 seconds on HIGH until the cheese melts and the tortilla softens.

1 pound lean ground beef

1 medium-size onion, peeled and diced

2 cloves garlic, smashed and peeled

3 tablespoons extra-virgin olive oil

1 teaspoon ground cumin

½ teaspoon Mexican chili powder, or to taste

Kosher salt and freshly ground black pepper, to taste

1 (15-ounce) can black beans, drained and rinsed

¼ cup prepared salsa

1 (1-pound) bag triple-washed fresh baby spinach

1 recipe Flour Tortillas (page 80), kept warm, or 8 gluten-free corn tortillas,
    moistened and warmed in the microwave oven until pliable

6 to 8 ounces Monterey Jack cheese, grated

1. In a large skillet over medium-high heat, cook the ground beef, stirring occasionally, until browned. Remove the beef from the skillet and set it aside.

2. In the same skillet, sauté the onion and garlic in the oil over medium-high heat, stirring frequently, until the onion is translucent and the garlic is fragrant, about 6 minutes. Add the cumin, chili powder, salt, and pepper, and stir. Add the beans and salsa and stir gently, taking care not to smash the beans. Lower the heat to medium and cook until heated through.

3. In a separate skillet, place the spinach and add a splash of water. Cover and cook over medium-high heat until just wilted, only a minute or 2. Remove from the heat.

4. Open the first tortilla, sprinkle a bit of cheese over the top, and then spoon about one-sixth of the beef mixture horizontally across the center of the tortilla. Top with some wilted spinach and more grated cheese. Fold in the sides of the tortilla, and roll away from you until the burrito is sealed. Press down lightly.

5. Repeat with the remaining tortillas. Microwave each tortilla on HIGH for about 45 seconds, or until the cheese is fully melted and has sealed the burrito closed. Allow the burrito to sit briefly before serving, to allow it to become a bit firm and more stable.

Shoestring Savings

On a shoestring: $1.74 each

If you bought it: $3.84 each (frozen)

Beef Taquitos

MAKES 4 TO 6 SERVINGS

Time Estimate: 13 minutes active time, 12 minutes inactive time

Can be doubled or halved easily

....

Taquitos are like a spin-off of burritos made with corn tortillas. Typically fried, this baked version saves you on ingredients (deep-frying requires a whole lot of oil), mess, bother—and calories, too! They make a great lunch, light dinner, or fun appetizer.

1 pound lean ground beef

1 medium-size onion, peeled and diced

2 cloves garlic, smashed and peeled

3 tablespoons extra-virgin olive oil, plus more for brushing

1 teaspoon ground cumin

½ teaspoon Mexican chili powder, or to taste

Kosher salt and freshly ground black pepper, to taste

8 gluten-free corn tortillas, moistened and warmed in the microwave oven
   until pliable

6 to 8 ounces Monterey Jack cheese, grated

Prepared salsa and sour cream, for serving

1. Preheat your oven to 400°F. Line a rimmed baking sheet with nonstick aluminum foil or unbleached parchment paper and set it aside.

2. In a large skillet over medium-high heat, cook the ground beef, stirring occasionally, until browned. Remove the beef from the skillet and set it aside.

3. In the same skillet, sauté the onion and garlic in the oil over medium-high heat, stirring frequently, until the onion is translucent and the garlic is fragrant, about 6 minutes. Add the beef, cumin, chili powder, salt, and pepper, and stir.

4. Open the first tortilla, scatter a bit of cheese over the top, and then spoon about one-eighth of the beef mixture on top of the cheese, leaving about an inch border around the perimeter of the tortilla. Top with more grated cheese evenly over the beef mixture. Roll the tortilla tightly from one side to the other. Place, seam side down, on the prepared baking sheet. Repeat with the rest of the tortillas. Brush the tops of the *taquitos* with olive oil.

5. Bake the *taquitos* in the center of the oven until the cheese is melted and the *taquitos* are lightly browned, about 12 minutes. Serve immediately with prepared salsa and sour cream.

Shoestring Savings

On a shoestring: 83¢/serving

If you bought it: $3.83/serving (frozen)

Pesto Chicken Pizza

MAKES 4 SERVINGS

Time Estimate: 20 minutes active time, 20 minutes inactive time
Can be doubled or halved easily

···

Pesto doesn't have to be made with basil. Try an equal amount of an alternative herb, such as parsley, or a leafy, flavorful green, such as arugula.

It's even faster to put together this dinner if you make your pesto ahead of time and store it in the refrigerator in an airtight container, or freeze portions of it in an ice cube tray for anytime use.

1 recipe Yeasted Refrigerator Pizza Dough (page 63)

¼ cup pine nuts

3 cups roughly chopped fresh basil leaves

4 cloves garlic, peeled

1 cup grated Parmigiano-Reggiano

½ cup extra-virgin olive oil

2 cups cubed gluten free rotisserie chicken

1 dry pint (2 cups) grape tomatoes, halved

6 ounces feta cheese, crumbled

1. Preheat your oven to 425°F. Place a pizza stone (or an overturned rimmed baking sheet, if you don't have one) in the oven as it heats.

2. Divide the pizza dough into two equal portions and roll each into a ball. Set the dough aside, covered loosely with a wet towel.

3. Take one piece of dough, and place it on a lightly floured piece of unbleached parchment paper. Dust the dough lightly with flour, cover with another sheet of unbleached parchment paper, and roll into a 12-inch round. Remove the top sheet of parchment paper. Roll in the edges to create a crust, and pinch to secure. Repeat with the second ball of dough.

4. Place each crust, one at a time, each still on a piece of parchment paper, on the hot pizza stone or overturned baking sheet. Bake for about 5 minutes, or until the crust begins to stiffen a bit, then remove it from the oven.

5. While the pizza crust is parbaking, make the pesto. In a dry skillet (preferably cast iron) over medium heat, toast the pine nuts gently, tossing frequently and taking care not to burn them, until fragrant and lightly browned, about 3 minutes. Remove the skillet from the heat and set it aside.

6. In the bowl of your food processor fitted with the steel blade, place the basil leaves, garlic, and grated Parmigiano-Reggiano cheese. Pulse until finely chopped. Add the toasted pine nuts, and pulse again to chop. Turn on the food processor and stream in the olive oil. Pulse until the pesto reaches your preferred consistency.

7. Divide the pesto between the two pizzas. Spread it with the back of a spoon into an even layer on the top of each pizza. Divide the chicken and tomatoes, followed by the crumbled feta cheese, between the two pizzas.

8. Place the pizzas, still on the parchment paper, on the pizza stone or overturned baking sheet in the oven. Bake until the cheese has melted and the tomatoes are wilting, about 7 minutes. Allow the cheese to set for a couple of minutes before slicing and serving.

Chapter 7

Shortcut Desserts

CAKES, PIES, COOKIES, AND BARS

Between the Twinkie-Style Cupcakes (page 154) and the Peanut Butter Cookies (page 181), both made with gluten-free yellow cake mix, a fabulous gluten-free dessert is always within reach. If you're looking for something a bit more sophisticated, try the Quick Chocolate Éclairs (page 160) for a bakery-style favorite that will impress the pants off those neighbors who are still stuck in that gluten-free-means-taste-free loop. The Chocolate Clafouti (page 163) can also be an impressive but deceptively easy change of pace, especially when you make individual portions.

The Chocolate Mousse Pie (page 177) takes no time to make and is plenty decadent. It does need to be refrigerated until firm, but it can be made a few days ahead of time with excellent results. And instead of fussing with individual drop cookies, try bar cookies. The time savings is pretty substantial. Read on for even more ideas for a sweet finish to any meal, even on a weeknight.

- Crazy Cake
- Almond Butter Brownie Bites
- Cheesecake Cookies
- Twinkie-Style Cupcakes
- "Key" Lime Pie Squares
- Classic British Flapjacks

- Quick Chocolate Éclairs
- Chocolate Clafouti
- Magic Bars
- No-Bake Cheesecake
- Dairy-Free Chocolate Peanut Butter Fudge
- Dairy-Free Coconut Chocolate Chip Cookie Bars
- Vanilla Wafer Bars
- Ho Ho–Style Cake
- Chocolate Mousse Pie with Sugar Cookie Crust
- Dairy-Free Baked Rice Pudding
- Peanut Butter Cookies
- Thumbprint Cookies
- Lemon Crinkle Cookies
- Apple Brown Betty

Crazy Cake

Time Estimate: 10 minutes active time, 25 minutes inactive time
MAKES ONE 9-INCH CAKE
Can be doubled or halved easily

⋯⋯⋯⋯⋯⋯⋯⋯⋯⋯⋯⋯⋯⋯⋯⋯⋯⋯⋯⋯⋯⋯⋯⋯⋯⋯⋯⋯

Crazy cake is not really so crazy. It's a Depression-era special, when butter and eggs were out of reach for many. Necessity is, indeed, the mother of invention. This is a nice chocolate cake that couldn't be simpler. When you make it, you'll take one look at the batter and you'll be afraid that it's not going to amount to anything when it grows up. But it will! And it's the dessert to make when you're craving chocolate cake but have run out of butter or milk, or when you're baking dairy-free.

1½ cups (210 g) high-quality all-purpose gluten-free flour

¾ teaspoon xanthan gum (omit if your blend already contains it)

1 cup (200 g) sugar

½ teaspoon kosher salt

1 teaspoon baking soda

¼ cup (20 g) natural unsweetened cocoa powder

6 tablespoons (84 g) vegetable oil

1 tablespoon white wine vinegar

1 teaspoon pure vanilla extract

1 cup water, at room temperature

1. Preheat your oven to 350°F. Grease a 9-inch square or round baking pan and set it aside.

2. In a large bowl, place the flour, xanthan gum, sugar, salt, baking soda, and cocoa powder, and whisk well. Add the oil, vinegar, vanilla, and water, mixing well after each addition.

3. Pour the batter into the prepared pan and place in the center of the preheated oven. Bake for 25 to 30 minutes, or until the cake has begun to pull away from the sides of the pan and a toothpick inserted into the center comes out clean.

4. Let cool in the pan for a few minutes, and then transfer to a wire rack to cool completely. Go crazy.

Almond Butter Brownie Bites

Time Estimate: 10 minutes active time, 12 minutes inactive time

MAKES 24 MINI MUFFINS

Can be doubled or halved easily

....

My celiac son comes home from school sometimes, and thinking he's being coy, announces that one of his classmates had something special for lunch that day. I get the hint, and put it on the list. These little brownie bites were my answer to the sort of packaged mini muffin he just had to have. And with the addition of almond butter to these mini muffins, he's getting more protein than anything else. Win-win.

1 cup plus 3 tablespoons (304 g) smooth no-stir almond butter

1 teaspoon pure vanilla extract

2 extra-large eggs, at room temperature, lightly beaten

7 tablespoons (61 g) high-quality all-purpose gluten-free flour

Scant ½ teaspoon xanthan gum (omit if your blend already contains it)

1. Preheat your oven to 350°F. Grease or line a standard 24-cup mini muffin tin and set it aside.

2. In a large, microwave-safe bowl, place the almond butter. Microwave for 45 seconds at 50 percent power. Remove from the microwave and stir the almond butter until smooth. Microwave for another 45 seconds at 50 percent power, if necessary to melt the almond butter.

3. Once the almond butter is smooth, allow to cool slightly. Add the vanilla and stir. Add the eggs, flour, and xanthan gum, mixing well after each addition.

4. Fill the prepared muffin cups about three-quarters of the way full. Bake the brownie bites in the center of the oven until they are mostly firm to the touch, about 12 minutes. Allow to cool completely in the tin before serving.

Shoestring Savings

On a shoestring: 23¢ each, or $2.74 for 12

If you bought it: 67¢ each, or $8 for 12

Cheesecake Cookies

Time Estimate: 7 minutes active time, 8 minutes inactive time
MAKES 2 DOZEN COOKIES
Can be doubled or halved easily

....

Soft, warm, and sinfully tasty, these cookies are the answer to the I-wish-I-had-a-piece-of-cheesecake-but-I'm-short-on-patience conundrum. Not only do they not need time to set up like a cheesecake does, but with only five ingredients, they go from fantasy to reality in a mere 15 minutes flat. As written, the recipe makes a relatively thin but soft cookie. For a thicker and more cakelike cookie, add one additional extra-large egg.

1 (16-ounce) box gluten-free yellow cake mix, or 1 recipe Make-Your-Own Vanilla
    Cake Mix (page 193)
8 ounces mascarpone cheese or cream cheese, at room temperature
4 tablespoons (56 g) unsalted butter, at room temperature
½ teaspoon pure vanilla extract
1 extra-large egg, at room temperature, beaten

1. Preheat your oven to 350°F. Line a rimmed baking sheet with unbleached parchment paper and set it aside.

2. In a large bowl, place the cake mix, and whisk to break up any lumps. Add the mascarpone, butter, vanilla, and egg, mixing well after each addition. The dough will be thick.

3. Drop the dough by rounded teaspoonfuls onto the prepared baking sheet, 1 inch apart. Bake the cookies in the center of the oven for 8 to 10 minutes, or until they are just beginning to brown on the underside and the edges. Allow to cool until set on the baking sheet. Transfer to a wire rack to cool completely.

Twinkie-Style Cupcakes

Time estimate: 15 minutes active time, 22 minutes inactive time
MAKES 1 DOZEN CUPCAKES
Can be doubled or halved easily

....

The rumors of the demise of the Twinkie have been greatly exaggerated. Hostess may not be able to make Twinkies forever, given its recent spate of financial troubles, but you can have a gluten-free version that would make the real thing jealous. And it's as easy as making vanilla cupcakes from a mix. This recipe makes cupcakes, rather than little Twinkie-shaped submarines, for the sake of time and convenience. (For a more authentic Twinkie shape, you can use a Norpro "cream canoe" pan. But for me, it's all just a delivery system for the filling.) I like to serve these upside down, so you can see the filling eagerly poking up through the holes.

CAKE

1 (16-ounce) box gluten-free yellow cake mix, or 1 recipe Make-Your-Own Vanilla
    Cake Mix (page 193)
2 tablespoons (24 g) vegetable shortening, melted and cooled
2 tablespoons (28 g) unsalted butter, melted and cooled
⅔ cup water, at room temperature
5 ounces egg whites (from about 4 extra-large eggs), at room temperature

FILLING

8 ounces (about 225 g) marshmallow crème
½ cup (96 g) vegetable shortening, melted and cooled
⅓ cup (38 g) confectioners' sugar
½ teaspoon pure vanilla extract

1. Preheat your oven to 325°F. Grease or line a standard 12-cup muffin tin, and set it aside.

2. Place the cake mix in a large bowl and whisk a bit to break up any lumps. Add the shortening, butter, and water, and mix well. The batter will be thick.

3. In the bowl of your stand mixer fitted with the whisk attachment, beat the egg whites until stiff but not dry.

4. Scrape half the egg whites into the bowl of batter and fold in gently. Add the remaining egg whites and fold gently until only a few white streaks remain.

5. Fill the wells of the prepared muffin tin about three-quarters of the way full. Place the tin in the center of the preheated oven and bake for about 22 minutes, rotating the pan once during baking. The cupcakes are done when a toothpick inserted into the center of the middle muffin comes out nearly clean. Allow the cupcakes to cool in the pan.

6. While the cupcakes are cooling, make the filling. In the bowl of your stand mixer fitted with the paddle attachment, place the marshmallow crème and shortening. Beat on medium speed to mix well. Add the confectioners' sugar and vanilla, and beat on high speed until fluffy. Transfer the filling mixture to a pastry bag fitted with a small "Bismarck tube" pastry tip. (The Ateco 230 tip is a great choice.)

7. Once the cupcakes have cooled, invert them onto a piece of parchment paper. With a wooden skewer or large toothpick, make four holes in the underside of each cupcake, and wiggle the tip around a bit to create space for filling. Insert the pastry tip into each of the holes, and pipe in some filling (as much or as little as you like). Repeat with the remaining cupcakes.

Shoestring Savings

On a shoestring: 44¢ each

If you bought it: $2.13 each

"Key" Lime Pie Squares

Time Estimate: 10 minutes active time,
25 minutes inactive time (plus refrigeration)

MAKES 24 BARS

Can be doubled or halved easily

....

Okay, so these aren't *Key* Lime Pie Squares, but they do taste remarkably like the real thing. Juicing Key limes is neither quick nor easy. They are so very tiny, and not a one of them provides much juice. You need about 2 pounds of them to make 1 cup of juice. To avoid the trouble, they've been replaced here with the juice of two regular limes and two to three lemons for a total of 1 cup. Much easier. But remember to use freshly squeezed juice! Most bottled lemon and lime juices are painfully sour. Buy a simple citrus reamer to make juicing easy, and it's done in no time.

7 to 8 ounces crunchy gluten-free cookies (such as Schär shortbread cookies,
     or the Vanilla Wafer Bars on page 172)
¼ teaspoon kosher salt
8 tablespoons (112 g) unsalted butter, melted and cooled
¼ cup (50 g) sugar
1 cup lemon-lime juice (juice of 2 limes and 2 to 3 lemons to make 1 cup of
     juice)
4 extra-large egg yolks, at room temperature, lightly beaten
2 (14-ounce) cans sweetened condensed milk

1. Preheat your oven to 375°F. Grease the bottom of a 9-inch square baking pan and line it with unbleached parchment paper that overhangs two opposite sides of the pan. Grease the paper, and then place another, crisscrossed sheet of parchment paper on top that overhangs the other two sides. Set the pan aside.

2. To make the crust, place the cookies and ⅛ teaspoon of the salt in the bowl of your food processor and pulse until finely ground. Transfer the cookie crumbs to a large bowl, add the butter and sugar, and mix well. The mixture should hold when pressed together.

3. Scrape the cookie mixture into the prepared baking dish. Press the crust evenly into a single layer in the bottom of the pan. Cover and place the pan in the freezer while making the filling.

4. To make the filling, place the lemon-lime juice, egg yolks, condensed milk, and remaining ⅛ teaspoon of salt in a large bowl and whisk until smooth.

5. Remove the baking dish from the freezer and pour the filling into the chilled crust. Tap the pie plate flat on the counter a few times to break any air bubbles that have formed in the filling.

6. Place the pie in the center of the oven and bake for about 25 minutes, or until the filling is set and the edges have begun to caramelize. Remove from the oven and allow to cool to room temperature.

7. Cover the pie and refrigerate it for 2 hours or up to overnight, before slicing into twenty-four bars and serving—or freeze it for about 45 minutes to speed things up. Serve chilled, with a lime wedge and a dollop of whipped cream.

Classic British Flapjacks

Time Estimate: 10 minutes active time, 20 minutes inactive time
MAKES 16 PIECES
Can be doubled or halved easily

....

To my American ears, a flapjack is a pancake. But in the United Kingdom, flapjacks are a bar cookie made with oats, butter, brown sugar, and Lyle's golden syrup. Lyle's is a thick and smooth syrup, similar to honey, but it doesn't crystallize like honey and it has really nice depth of flavor. It might very well be for sale at your local market as it is in mine, and you just never noticed it before.

2½ cups (250 g) gluten-free old-fashioned rolled oats
8 tablespoons (112 g) unsalted butter, chopped
½ cup (109 g) packed light brown sugar
¼ cup Lyle's golden syrup or honey

1. Preheat your oven to 350°F. Grease the bottom of a 9-inch square baking pan and line it with unbleached parchment paper that overhangs two opposite sides of the pan. Grease the paper, and then place another, crisscrossed sheet of parchment paper on top that overhangs the other two sides. Set the pan aside.

2. Place the oats in a blender or food processor, and grind or pulse until the oats are more processed by about half.

3. Place the butter, sugar, and golden syrup in a medium-size saucepan and cook, stirring constantly, over medium heat until the butter and sugar have melted. Remove the pan from the heat and pour in the processed oats. Stir until well mixed. Scrape the mixture into the prepared pan, and with a wet spatula, press it evenly into the bottom of the pan.

4. Place in the center of the oven and bake for 15 minutes, or until the edges are just beginning to brown. The flapjacks will seem soft and won't yet hold together well. Remove the pan from the oven and immediately score the contents into sixteen squares, while the flapjacks are still warm. If you don't cut into the flapjacks while they are still warm, they will be too brittle to slice once they are cool.

5. Let cool completely in the pan, and then, grabbing by the overhanging parchment paper, remove the flapjacks from the pan. Place on a cutting board, and with a very sharp knife, cut the flapjacks along the scored lines. They will keep for about 5 days in an airtight container at room temperature.

Quick Chocolate Éclairs

Time Estimate: 20 minutes active time, 25 minutes inactive time
MAKES 12 TO 15 ÉCLAIRS
Can be doubled or halved easily

....

Éclairs are not nearly the sticky wicket you might think, but they do tend to take a bit of time. This quick version shaves off time in two important ways. First, the cream filling is made using Bird's Custard Powder, a British phenomenon created by Mr. Bird, who wanted to make custard for his wife, who was egg-free. The result was a powder not unlike cornstarch that thickens into custard when you add sugar and milk to it, and warm it either in the microwave or on the stovetop. Éclair filling in a snap.

The second time-saver is using a blender to smooth the light, French-style choux pastry ingredients rather than mixing by hand like an overworked milkmaid until the dough becomes smooth after adding the eggs. I've made it both ways, and I can't taste the difference between the traditional method and the quick one.

FILLING

2 tablespoons (35 g) Bird's Custard Powder

2 tablespoons (24 g) sugar

3½ cups milk (low-fat is fine, nonfat is not)

PASTRY

1 cup milk (low-fat is fine, nonfat is not)

4 tablespoons (56 g) unsalted butter

Dash (⅛ teaspoon) of kosher salt

1 cup (140 g) high-quality all-purpose gluten-free flour

½ teaspoon xanthan gum (omit if your blend already contains it)

4 extra-large eggs, at room temperature, beaten

CHOCOLATE TOPPING

5 ounces semisweet chocolate, chopped

3 tablespoons (36 g) vegetable shortening

1. First, make the filling. In a medium, heat-safe bowl, whisk together the custard powder and sugar. Add 2 tablespoons of milk from the 3½ cups, and mix into a smooth paste.

2. In a medium-size, heavy-bottomed saucepan, heat the rest of the 3½ cups of milk until simmering. Remove the pan from the heat and pour the hot milk slowly over the custard paste, whisking constantly. Pour the mixture back into the saucepan and cook over medium heat, stirring constantly, until thickened, about 5 minutes. Remove from the heat and allow to cool.

3. While the filling is cooling, make the pastries. Preheat your oven to 425°F. Line rimmed baking sheets with unbleached parchment paper and set them aside.

4. Cook the milk, butter, and salt in a large saucepan until the butter is melted and the mixture begins to boil. Remove the pan from the heat, add the flour and xanthan gum, and stir vigorously. Return to the heat and continue to stir vigorously for about 3 minutes, until the mixture begins to pull away from the sides of the pan and comes together in a ball. A thin film will form on the bottom of the pan. Remove from the heat and allow the mixture to cool for about 3 minutes.

5. Transfer half the dough to a blender or food processor. Pour the beaten eggs on top and then add the rest of the dough. Pulse until the mixture is smooth and uniformly well blended.

6. Transfer the dough from the blender to a pastry bag fitted with a large, plain tip. Pipe the dough in lines about 4 inches long apiece onto the prepared baking sheets, spacing the pastries 2 inches apart from one another.

7. Bake the éclairs in the center of the oven for 10 minutes. Turn down the temperature to 375°F, and finish baking for about another 15 minutes, until pale golden. Allow the pastries to cool completely on the baking sheets.

8. To make the chocolate topping, place the chopped chocolate and shortening in a medium-size, microwave-safe bowl. Place the bowl in the microwave and heat for 45 seconds at 70 percent power. Stir the mixture, and heat again for 45 seconds at 70 percent power. Stir and repeat if necessary until all the chocolate is melted and smooth. Set aside to cool briefly.

9. Once the éclairs are cool, transfer the filling mixture to a pastry bag fitted with a small "Bismarck tube" pastry tip. (The Ateco 230 tip is a great choice.) Pierce the first éclair with the pastry tip and pipe the filling inside (as much or as little as you like). Repeat with the remaining éclairs.

10. Pour the chocolate topping over each filled éclair, and spread it evenly over the top. Allow the éclairs to sit at room temperature until the chocolate sets.

VARIATION: Once you've mastered this dough, try making it into round puffs to make profiteroles. Slice the cooled puffs in half horizontally, fill with ice cream, and drizzle with the chocolate topping.

Shoestring Savings

On a shoestring: 58¢ each

If you bought it: $2.75 each

Chocolate Clafouti

Time Estimate: 10 minutes active time, 25 minutes inactive time
MAKES 4 SERVINGS
Can be doubled or halved easily

....

Sweet clafouti is such a treat. It's similar to a soufflé, but much less temperamental and intimidating. Make individual servings and you have an elegant and rich dessert that will impress any of the self-proclaimed foodies in your life.

Unsalted butter for greasing ramekins
½ cup plus 1 tablespoon (79 g) high-quality all-purpose gluten-free flour
¼ teaspoon xanthan gum (omit if your blend already contains it)
½ cup (109 g) packed light brown sugar
3 tablespoons (36 g) granulated sugar
1 teaspoon pure vanilla extract
4 extra-large eggs, at room temperature, lightly beaten
2 cups heavy whipping cream, at room temperature
2 ounces semisweet or dark chocolate, chopped
2 ounces white chocolate, chopped

1. Preheat your oven to 400°F. Grease well with unsalted butter four 1-cup ramekins (or one 4- to 6-cup ramekin) and set them aside.

2. In a large bowl, place the ½ cup of the flour and the xanthan gum, brown sugar, and granulated sugar, and whisk well. Add the vanilla, eggs, and cream, and mix well.

3. In a separate small bowl, place both kinds of chopped chocolate and the reserved tablespoon of flour, and toss to coat the chocolate in the flour. Add the chocolate to the cream mixture and stir well.

4. Divide the batter evenly among the prepared ramekins. Place all four ramekins on a large rimmed baking sheet. Bake until puffed and light golden brown on top, about 25 minutes. Serve warm.

Magic Bars

Time Estimate: 10 minutes active time, 20 minutes inactive time

MAKES 16 BARS

Can be doubled or halved easily

....

If you've never had one form or another of a magic bar, you might be surprised by how pleasantly chewy the cereal tastes once it's been softened and then baked. It makes these bars a real treat and a sweet alternative to traditional blondies. Feel free to substitute any sort of chips for the white chocolate.

1 cup (140 g) high-quality all-purpose gluten-free flour

½ teaspoon xanthan gum (omit if your blend already contains it)

½ teaspoon baking powder

Dash (⅛ teaspoon) of baking soda

½ teaspoon kosher salt

1 cup (218 g) packed light brown sugar

6 tablespoons (84 g) unsalted butter, at room temperature

2 extra-large eggs, at room temperature, lightly beaten

1 tablespoon pure vanilla extract

1 cup (about 75 g) crushed, flaky gluten-free cereal of choice (gluten-free corn
   flakes work well)

⅔ cup (112 g) white chocolate chips

1. Preheat your oven to 350°F. Grease a 9-inch square baking pan and set the pan aside.

2. In a large bowl, place the flour, xanthan gum, baking powder, baking soda, salt, and brown sugar, and whisk until well mixed, making sure to break up any lumps in the brown sugar. Add the butter and mix until the batter is crumbly and moist. Add the eggs and vanilla, and beat until the batter is smooth and shiny.

3. In a separate, medium-size bowl, place the crushed cereal and white chocolate chips and toss to mix. Add the cereal and chip mixture to the batter and mix gently to fold it in until it is evenly distributed throughout the batter. Scrape the batter into the prepared pan and spread into an even layer with a wet spatula.

4. Place in the center of the oven and bake, rotating once during baking, for 20 to 25 minutes, or until the edges of the bars are beginning to brown and they are just set in the middle. Let cool completely in the pan before slicing into sixteen squares. Serve chilled or at room temperature.

Shoestring Savings

On a shoestring: $3.36/dozen

If you bought it: $9.26/dozen

No-Bake Cheesecake

Time Estimate: 15 minutes active time, 30 minutes in freezer until set
SERVES 6
Can be doubled easily

··

I like Cool Whip just as much as the next person, but it has such a distinctive flavor that a cheesecake made with it tastes to me like nothing more than the famous whipped topping itself. I prefer cheesecake to taste like, well, cheesecake, even if it's a quick, no-bake variety. If you feel similarly, or even if you're just curious, give this version a try. How can you go wrong with cheesecake?

7 to 8 ounces crunchy gluten-free cookies (such as Schär shortbread cookies,
     or the Vanilla Wafer Bars, page 172)
Dash (⅛ teaspoon) kosher salt
8 tablespoons (112 g) unsalted butter, melted and cooled
¼ cup (50 g) granulated sugar
⅓ cup heavy cream, chilled
⅓ cup (38 g) confectioners' sugar
4 ounces cream cheese, at room temperature
4 ounces mascarpone cheese, at room temperature, or 4 ounces of another
     cream cheese
Juice of 1 medium-size lemon (about 4 tablespoons)

1. Grease a 9-inch pie plate and set it aside.

2. Place the cookies and the salt in the bowl of your food processor and pulse until finely ground. Transfer the cookie crumbs to a large bowl, add the butter and granulated sugar to the bowl, and mix well. The mixture should hold when pressed together.

3. Scrape the cookie mixture into the prepared pie plate and press it evenly into the bottom and up the sides of the pan, stopping just short of the lip of the plate. Cover and place the plate in the freezer while making the filling.

4. In the bowl of your stand mixer fitted with the whisk attachment, whip the heavy cream on medium-high speed until it forms soft peaks, adding the confectioners' sugar as it whips. Scrape the whipped cream into a separate large bowl.

5. Fit your mixer with the paddle attachment, place the cream cheese, mascarpone, and lemon juice in the mixer bowl and beat until light and fluffy. Remove the bowl from the mixer and fold the whipped cream gently into the cream cheese mixture.

6. Remove the crust from the freezer and pour the filling into it. Smooth with an offset spatula. Carefully cover the cheesecake with plastic wrap and freeze for about 30 minutes, or until firm. Store in the refrigerator until ready to use. Serve chilled.

Shoestring Savings

On a shoestring: $1.21/serving

If you bought it: $4.22/serving (frozen)

Dairy-Free Chocolate Peanut Butter Fudge

Time Estimate: 15 minutes active time, inactive time for refrigeration
MAKES 16 PIECES
Can be doubled or halved easily

....

The secret to this fudge is dairy-free sweetened condensed milk. And the secret to making dairy-free sweetened condensed milk is cooking it long enough. It takes at least 10 minutes for the mixture of coconut milk (canned, not the kind you drink) and sugar to thicken properly and be up to the job of setting up fudge. If you're unsure of the way the sweetened condensed coconut milk should look before it can be considered ready, see the photos on my blog in the post for Dairy-Free White Chocolate Fudge: http://glutenfreeonashoestring.com/dairy-free-white-chocolate-fudge-think-garnish-for-valentines-day/. It has to be that thick.

2 (14-ounce) cans coconut milk (regular, not low-fat)
½ cup (100 g) sugar
26 ounces (720 g) dairy-free semisweet chocolate, chopped (chips will do)
1 teaspoon pure vanilla extract
1 tablespoon (14 g) virgin coconut oil or vegetable shortening
Dash (⅛ teaspoon) of kosher salt
1½ cups (384 g) natural no-stir peanut butter

1. Grease the bottom of an 8-inch square baking pan and line it with unbleached parchment paper that overhangs the opposite sides of the pan. Grease the paper, and then place another, crisscrossed sheet of parchment paper on top that also overhangs the other two sides. Set the pan aside.

2. In a medium-size saucepan over medium-high heat, bring the coconut milk and sugar to a boil. Continue to boil, stirring constantly, until the mixture is reduced by about half, the milk is thick and it has begun to turn light amber in color as the sugar begins to caramelize, about 10 minutes. While it is reducing, the milk will bubble quite a lot at first, but will not overflow as long as you keep stirring.

3. After most of the water has evaporated, the mixture will become thick enough to coat the back of a spoon. Continue to cook until reduced a bit further. Remove the pan from the heat once the mixture is about as thick as traditional condensed milk.

4. Add the chocolate, vanilla, coconut oil, and salt to the saucepan, and stir vigorously until the chocolate is melted and the mixture is smooth. Add the peanut butter to the mixture and stir until well integrated.

5. Pour the batter into the prepared pan and shake until it is spread in an even layer. Bang the pan flat on the table a couple of times to ensure that there are no trapped air bubbles.

6. Place the pan in the refrigerator and chill until set, at least 2 hours and up to overnight. Once the fudge seems to be set, lift it from the pan, using the over-hanging sheets of parchment paper, and slice it into sixteen pieces with a large, wet knife. Serve chilled.

Shoestring Savings

On a shoestring: 58¢/piece

If you bought it: $1.66/piece

Dairy-Free Coconut Chocolate Chip Cookie Bars

Time Estimate: 10 minutes active time, 22 minutes inactive time

MAKES 24 BARS

Can be doubled or halved easily

....

You can make these into individual drop cookies, but cookie bars are so much quicker! Virgin coconut oil has a very subtle coconut flavor that makes it ideal for this sort of cookie. Here, the flavor is amplified by unsweetened coconut chips, which are thick curls of coconut that don't have any of that stringy texture that you sometimes get with shredded coconut. They taste great, and don't look half bad, either.

Be sure to use unrefined virgin coconut oil in this recipe, which is a solid white, thick paste at room temperature. Melt it by placing it in a microwave-safe bowl and zapping it on HIGH for about 30 seconds, and then stirring it.

2¼ cups (315 g) high-quality all-purpose gluten-free flour

1¼ teaspoons xanthan gum (omit if your blend already contains it)

½ teaspoon kosher salt

1 teaspoon baking powder

¼ teaspoon baking soda

1¼ cups (273 g) packed light brown sugar

¼ cup (50 g) granulated sugar

8 ounces dairy-free semisweet chocolate chips

1½ cups (120 g) unsweetened coconut chips

½ cup (112 g) virgin coconut oil, melted and cooled

2 extra-large eggs, at room temperature, beaten

1 tablespoon pure vanilla extract

1. Preheat your oven to 325°F. Line a rimmed baking sheet with unbleached parchment paper and set it aside.

2. In a large bowl, place the flour, xanthan gum, salt, baking powder, baking soda, brown sugar, and granulated sugar, and whisk well. Place the chocolate and

coconut chips in a separate, medium-size bowl, add a tablespoon of the dry ingredients to the bowl, and toss to coat. Set the chips aside.

3. Create a well in the center of the dry ingredients and add the coconut oil, eggs one at a time, and vanilla, beating well after each addition.

4. Stir the chips and reserved dry ingredients into the cookie dough until they are evenly distributed. The dough will be thick.

5. Transfer the dough to the prepared baking sheet, and press it into an even layer with wet hands. Place the bars in the center of the oven and bake until they are just beginning to brown around the edges, about 22 minutes. Remove the pan from the oven and allow the bars to cool in the pan until solid and cool to the touch. Slice into twenty-four pieces and serve. Freeze any leftovers in a freezer-safe container.

Vanilla Wafer Bars

Time Estimate: 10 minutes active time, 25 minutes inactive time

MAKES 16 BARS

Can be doubled or halved easily

....

You can make this recipe, my gluten-free version of the little round, snappy vanilla wafer cookies, as rounds, as I explain on my blog: http://glutenfreeonashoe string.com/nilla-wafers/. Or, you can make them the Quick and Easy way, into bars. These taste just as you remember them. In fact, that deep vanilla flavor is so pitch perfect, you'll think you pulled them right out of the brown waxed paper bag sitting in that familiar yellow box.

1⅓ cups (187 g) high-quality all-purpose gluten-free flour

½ teaspoon xanthan gum (omit if your blend already contains it)

½ teaspoon baking powder

Dash (⅛ teaspoon) of baking soda

½ teaspoon kosher salt

8 tablespoons (112 g) unsalted butter, at room temperature

½ cup (109 g) packed light brown sugar

1 extra-large egg, at room temperature, lightly beaten

4 teaspoons pure vanilla extract

2 tablespoons milk, at room temperature (any milk will do)

1. Preheat your oven to 325°F. Grease an 8-inch square baking pan, line it with unbleached parchment paper, and grease it again. Set the pan aside.

2. In the bowl of your stand mixer, place the flour, xanthan gum, baking powder, baking soda, and salt, and whisk by hand until well combined. Secure the mixer's paddle attachment, and with the mixer on low speed, add the butter, brown sugar, egg, vanilla, and milk, one ingredient at a time. The batter should be thick.

3. Scrape the dough with a spatula into the prepared baking pan. Wet the spatula and smooth the top of the dough in an even layer with no bits sticking up.

4. Place the pan in the center of your oven and bake until the dough is a nice, uniform brown color, as you would expect from boxed vanilla wafer cookies, about 25 minutes. Rotate once during baking.

5. Let cool in the pan until solid and slice into sixteen bars. Store leftovers in the freezer.

Shoestring Savings

On a shoestring: $2.40/dozen

If you bought it: $5.64/dozen

Ho Ho–Style Cake

Time Estimate: 25 minutes active time, 20 minutes inactive time
MAKES ONE 2-LAYER CAKE
Can be doubled or halved somewhat easily

....

This cake is one of my favorites, as it's the quickest and easiest straight line to a gluten-free Ho-Ho–type treat. Forget all that fooling around involved in rolling a thin sheet cake without cracking it. This cake is deep, chocolaty, and just plain good, but isn't tooth-achingly sweet. The filling is just stiff enough to remind you of Ho Hos or Yodels or Swiss rolls, whichever brand earned your childhood loyalty, and the chocolate topping cracks slightly under pressure. That might not be a desirable quality in a friend, but it's just perfect for this memorable treat. Make it even easier by making it in a single pan and using the filling as a topping with no chocolate shell.

CAKE

6 tablespoons (84 g) unsalted butter, at room temperature, plus more
    for greasing pans
1 cup (140 g) high-quality all-purpose gluten-free flour
½ teaspoon xanthan gum (omit if your blend already contains it)
2 tablespoons (10 g) natural unsweetened cocoa powder
½ teaspoon baking soda
¼ teaspoon kosher salt
6 ounces semisweet chocolate, chopped
1 cup (200 g) granulated sugar
½ teaspoon pure vanilla extract
4 extra-large eggs, at room temperature, beaten
¾ cup water, at room temperature, plus more by the tablespoon, if necessary

FILLING

1 packet (1 scant tablespoon) unflavored powdered gelatin
2 tablespoons cool water
2 cups heavy cream, chilled
3 tablespoons (22 g) confectioners' sugar

CHOCOLATE SHELL

10 ounces semisweet chocolate, chopped

6 tablespoons (84 g) vegetable shortening

1. Preheat your oven to 350°F. Grease with unsalted butter two 8-inch round cake pans. If you are concerned about the cake's having trouble coming out of the pans after baking, line the pans with unbleached parchment paper, and then grease the parchment paper. Set the pans aside.

2. To make the cake, place the flour, xanthan gum, cocoa powder, baking soda, and salt in a medium-size bowl, and whisk well.

3. In a separate large, microwave-safe bowl, place the chopped chocolate and 6 tablespoons of butter. Microwave on 50 percent power for 45 seconds at a time, stirring in between, until the chocolate and butter are melted and smooth. Allow to cool briefly.

4. Add the granulated sugar and vanilla to the chocolate mixture, and mix well. Add the eggs and water, and mix well. Add the dry ingredients to the chocolate mixture, and mix well. The batter should be pourable. If it seems too thick, thin it with another tablespoon or two of water.

5. Divide the batter between the prepared cake pans. Shake the pans from side to side to distribute the batter evenly. Smack the bottom of each pan against the counter to burst any air bubbles, and place both pans in the center of the oven. If there isn't enough room for both to be on the center rack, bake one at a time.

6. Bake for about 15 minutes, or until the cakes are just firm to the touch. Do not overbake. Remove the cakes from the oven and allow to cool at least 10 minutes in the pans before turning onto a wire rack to cool completely.

7. While the cakes are cooling, make the filling. Place the contents of the packet of powdered gelatin and the water in a small, microwave-safe bowl, and mix well. Allow to sit for a few moments until the gelatin swells. It will be lumpy. Microwave the gelatin mixture for 30 seconds on HIGH to liquefy it. Allow to cool for about 2 minutes.

8. In the bowl of a stand mixer fitted with the whisk attachment, beat the cream and confectioners' sugar on medium-high speed until soft peaks form. Add the slightly cooled gelatin mixture to the whipped cream and whisk again at high speed until the mixture has thickened, and it holds a stiff (but not dry) peak. Place the filling in the refrigerator to chill while the cakes finish cooling.

9. Once the cakes have cooled completely, place one cake top down on your serving plate. With an offset spatula, spread an even layer of filling about ½ inch thick over the entire surface of the cake. Top with the other cake.

10. To make the chocolate shell, place the chopped chocolate and shortening in a medium-size, microwave safe bowl. Place the bowl in the microwave and heat for 45 seconds at 50 percent power. Stir the mixture, and heat again for 45 seconds at 50 percent power. Stir and repeat if necessary until all the chocolate is melted and smooth.

11. Pour the chocolate mixture on the center of the top of the assembled cake. Spread carefully over the top, allowing it to drop down the sides. Allow the cake to sit at room temperature until the chocolate sets. Slice and serve.

Shoestring Savings

On a shoestring: 60¢/serving

If you bought it: $1.22/serving

Chocolate Mousse Pie with Sugar Cookie Crust

Time Estimate: 15 minutes active time, plus inactive time for refrigeration

MAKES ONE 9-INCH PIE

Can be doubled easily

....

This chocolate mousse pie can easily be made without a crust, or with a crumbled cookie crust like the one in No-Bake Cheesecake (page 166). Instead of a crumbled cookie crust, this has a softer crust made from, basically, one big cookie. It's the only thing that needs baking in the whole recipe, and this pie can be made a few days ahead of time, as the chocolate mousse is very stable. Keep it in the refrigerator, covered, until you're ready to serve it, and it will taste as good on the third day as it did on the first.

Remember that simple chocolate recipes such as chocolate mousse are only as good as the chocolate you use, so use the highest quality you can.

½ recipe Make-Your-Own Sugar Cookie Mix (page 201)

1 scant tablespoon (1 packet) unflavored powdered gelatin

2 tablespoons cool water

4 tablespoons (56 g) unsalted butter, at room temperature

12 ounces semisweet chocolate, chopped

1 teaspoon pure vanilla extract

2 cups heavy cream, chilled

2 tablespoons (14 g) confectioners' sugar

1. To make the cookie piecrust, prepare the cookie dough as indicated to make cookies, but press one half of the dough into the bottom and up the sides of a 9-inch nonstick or greased pie plate. Bake at 350°F for about 8 minutes, or until just set. Allow to cool completely before filling.

2. To make the mousse, place the contents of the packet of powdered gelatin and the 2 tablespoons of water in a small, microwave-safe bowl, and mix well. Allow to sit for a few moments until the gelatin swells. It will be lumpy. Microwave the gelatin mixture for 30 seconds on HIGH to liquefy it. Set the gelatin aside and allow to cool for about 2 minutes.

3. Place the butter and the chocolate in a large, microwave-safe bowl. Heat in the microwave at 70 percent power for 45 seconds at a time, stirring in between, until the chocolate and butter are melted and smooth. Add the vanilla and mix well. Set aside to cool a bit.

4. In the bowl of a stand mixer fitted with the whisk attachment, beat the cream and confectioners' sugar on medium-high speed until soft peaks form. Add the slightly cooled gelatin mixture to the whipped cream and whisk again at high speed until the mixture has thickened and holds a stiff (but not dry) peak. Carefully fold the cooled chocolate mixture into the whipped cream until only a few white streaks are still visible.

5. Pour the mousse into the pie shell and smooth the top with a cool, wet spatula. Refrigerate until set, 2 to 4 hours. You can speed up the process by placing the pie in the freezer for an hour. Serve chilled.

Shoestring Savings

On a shoestring: $9.50/pie

If you bought it: $25.00/pie

Dairy-Free Baked Rice Pudding

Time Estimate: 10 minutes active time, 1 hour inactive time

SERVES 4

Can be doubled or halved easily

....

Rice pudding shouldn't be difficult or particularly time-consuming to make on the stovetop. But it's easy to get distracted when the milk is simmering and then you have one unholy mess to clean up. That kind of cleanup runs any hope of a quick dessert right out of town. Solution: This rice pudding is baked in the oven. That means it requires little babysitting, so you can do other things while it's baking. Like make dinner, even.

Feel free to divide the pudding among four 3-cup soufflé dishes, instead of one main dish. Serve warm and soft or at room temperature and set.

¾ cup (144 g) uncooked Arborio (or other short-grain) rice

4 cups almond milk

2 cups low-fat coconut milk

2 tablespoons pure vanilla extract

6 tablespoons (42 g) confectioners' sugar

3 tablespoons (36 g) vegetable shortening

1 tablespoon ground cinnamon

1. Preheat your oven to 350°F.

2. Place the rice in a 10- to 12-cup ovenproof soufflé dish. Pour in the almond milk, coconut milk, and vanilla, add 4 tablespoons of the confectioners' sugar, and mix well. Cover the dish tightly with foil and bake for 30 minutes.

3. Take the dish out of the oven, remove the cover, and stir the rice. Add the vegetable shortening to the top and return the uncovered dish to the oven. Bake for another 20 minutes, or until the milk is mostly absorbed.

4. Open the oven and sprinkle the top of the pudding evenly with the remaining 2 tablespoons confectioners' sugar and the ground cinnamon. Continue to bake uncovered for another 10 minutes, or until the top is golden brown. Serve warm or at room temperature.

VARIATION: Replace the almond and coconut milks with 6 cups of low-fat or whole dairy milk, and the shortening with 3 tablespoons of unsalted butter, for a dairy version.

Peanut Butter Cookies

Time Estimate: 10 minutes active time, 11 minutes inactive time
MAKES 2 DOZEN COOKIES
Can be doubled or halved easily

··

I don't have to tell you that these soft and chewy peanut butter cookies bake up in a flash. You see a list of ingredients that short, and you know we're talking short and sweet. What you might not know yet, though, but will soon, is how the taste of peanut butter neither overwhelms nor disappoints in these hearty cookies. Perfect!

1 (16-ounce) box gluten-free yellow cake mix, or 1 recipe Make-Your-Own Vanilla
     Cake Mix (page 193)
1 cup (256 g) no-stir smooth peanut butter, such as Peanut Butter & Co. Smooth
     Operator
3 tablespoons (36 g) vegetable shortening
3 tablespoons (42 g) unsalted butter, at room temperature
2 extra-large eggs, at room temperature, lightly beaten
1 teaspoon pure vanilla extract

1. Preheat your oven to 350°F. Line a rimmed baking sheet with unbleached parchment paper and set it aside.

2. Place the cake mix in a large bowl, whisk to break up any lumps, and set it aside.

3. In a small, heavy-bottomed saucepan, place the peanut butter, shortening, and butter. Stir over medium heat until the ingredients are all melted and smooth. Remove from the heat and continue to stir to cool a bit.

4. Create a well in the center of the dry ingredients and pour in the peanut butter mixture. Mix well. Add the eggs and vanilla, and stir until incorporated.

5. Drop rounded teaspoons of cookie dough about 2 inches apart onto the prepared baking sheet.

6. Bake the cookies in the center of the oven for about 11 minutes, or until they appear cracked on top and are beginning to brown around the edges. Allow to cool until set on the baking sheet. Transfer to a wire rack to cool completely.

Shoestring Savings

On a shoestring: $2.46/dozen

If you bought it: $3.80/dozen

Thumbprint Cookies

Time Estimate: 15 minutes active time, 10 minutes inactive time
MAKES 2 DOZEN COOKIES
Can be doubled or halved easily

···

Have you ever made a nice-looking thumbprint cookie with your actual thumb? Near as I can tell, no one really has. I've tried making the thumbprint before and after baking, and neither creates a nice, round cup. Instead, I've found that using the bottom of a half-teaspoon measure is the perfect alternative. So if you can be troubled to wait around for 5 minutes of baking, press the bowl of the measuring spoon into the half-baked cookies, then return them to the oven, you shall be rewarded with just the right "thumbprint." And who doesn't like to make a good impression?

1½ cups (210 g) high-quality all-purpose gluten-free flour

¾ teaspoon xanthan gum (omit if your blend already contains it)

1¼ teaspoons baking powder

½ teaspoon kosher salt

½ cup (109 g) packed light brown sugar

8 tablespoons (112 g) unsalted butter, at room temperature

1 extra-large egg yolk, at room temperature, lightly beaten

1½ teaspoons pure vanilla extract

½ cup seedless fruit preserves or jam

1. Preheat your oven to 350°F. Line a rimmed baking sheet with unbleached parchment paper and set it aside.

2. In a large bowl, place the flour, xanthan gum, baking powder, salt, and brown sugar, and whisk to combine well, working out any lumps in the brown sugar. Add the butter, egg yolk, and vanilla, and mix well. Turn out the dough onto a piece of parchment paper (it will be kind of crumbly), and press it with your hands so that it holds together.

3. Divide the dough into twenty-four pieces. Roll each into a ball and place 1 inch apart on the prepared baking sheet. Freeze the dough on the baking sheet for about 10 minutes, or until it is firm.

4. Transfer the baking sheet to the oven and bake the cookies for 5 minutes. Remove the baking sheet from the oven. Wet the rounded side of a half-teaspoon measuring spoon, and press it gently but firmly into the center of each softened mound of dough. Add about ½ teaspoon of jam to each well and return the baking sheet to the oven. Bake the cookies for another 5 to 7 minutes, or until pale golden. Remove from the oven.

5. Allow the cookies to cool until firm on the baking sheet. Transfer to a wire rack to cool completely.

Shoestring Savings

On a shoestring: $1.00/serving

If you bought it: $2.22/serving

Lemon Crinkle Cookies

Time Estimate: 15 minutes active time, 10 minutes inactive time
MAKES 2 DOZEN COOKIES
Can be doubled or halved easily

....

These cookies are a riff on chocolate crinkle cookies, which are those pretty choco-late cookies with the crinkled appearance and the confectioners' sugar lining the cracks. They have a nice, tangy, lemony zing, and you'd never guess that they use a cake mix as their base. If you'd rather keep them even simpler, skip rolling the cookie dough in confectioners' sugar. They'll still be tangy-sweet, pretty little yel-low cookies.

1 (16-ounce) box gluten-free yellow cake mix, or 1 recipe Make-Your-Own Vanilla
   Cake Mix (page 193)
Zest of 1 lemon (about 1 tablespoon zest)
2 tablespoons (28 g) unsalted butter, melted and cooled
4 tablespoons (28 g) vegetable shortening, melted and cooled
2 tablespoons freshly squeezed lemon juice (juice of about ½ lemon)
2 extra-large eggs, at room temperature, beaten
About 1 cup (115 g) confectioners' sugar, for rolling

   1. Preheat your oven to 350°F. Line a rimmed baking sheet with unbleached parchment paper and set it aside.
   2. Place the cake mix and lemon zest in a large bowl and whisk to break up any lumps and to separate the pieces of lemon zest. Add the butter, shortening, lemon juice, and eggs, mixing well after each addition. The dough will be thick.
   3. Drop rounded teaspoons of dough about 1½ inches apart on the prepared baking sheet. Place in the freezer to chill for about 10 minutes, or until firm.
   4. Place the confectioners' sugar in a medium-size bowl. Remove the cookie dough from the freezer. Pick up the pieces of cookie dough one by one, and roll each into a ball. Place each ball of dough into the bowl of confectioners' sugar, toss to coat completely in sugar, and then place about 1½ inches apart on the prepared

baking sheet. Freeze the dough on the baking sheet for about 10 minutes, or until it is firm.

5. Bake the cookies in the center of the oven for 6 to 8 minutes, or until just beginning to brown on the underside and slightly on the edges. They will still be soft to the touch, but will become firm as they cool. Allow to cool until set on the baking sheet. Transfer to a wire rack to cool completely.

Apple Brown Betty

Time Estimate: 20 minutes active time
MAKES 4 SERVINGS
Can be doubled or halved easily

I've long found the prospect of an apple brown betty to be a comfort. Gently spiced, warm, and inviting, it's the perfect finish to any meal. And this version is super speedy quick, because it's made entirely on the stovetop. The filling can even be made ahead of time and stored in the refrigerator in an airtight container for up to 2 days. Just warm the refrigerated filling gently over low heat after making the topping, and serve as directed.

TOPPING

4 tablespoons (56 g) unsalted butter

2 cups fresh, coarsely ground gluten-free bread crumbs

½ teaspoon ground cinnamon, or more to taste

¼ teaspoon freshly grated nutmeg

½ cup (109 g) packed light brown sugar

FILLING

2 tablespoons (28 g) unsalted butter

4 large firm apples (Empire is a good choice), peeled, cored, and sliced thinly

2 tablespoons (24 g) granulated sugar

1. First, make the topping. In a medium-size skillet over medium-high heat, melt the butter until it begins to bubble. Add the bread crumbs and stir. Lower the heat to medium-low and cook slowly, stirring occasionally, until the bread crumbs are lightly browned, about 5 minutes. Add the cinnamon, nutmeg, and brown sugar, and stir until the sugar has melted into the bread crumbs. Remove the skillet from the heat and set it aside.

2. To make the filling, in a separate medium-size skillet over medium-high heat, melt the butter until it begins to bubble. Add the apples and granulated

sugar, and stir. Lower the heat to medium, cover the skillet, and cook, stirring occasionally, until the apples are softened (about 7 minutes, depending upon how thinly you have sliced the apples).

3. To assemble the dish, divide the warm filling among four dessert plates and then divide the topping evenly over the tops. Serve warm, with a scoop of vanilla ice cream.

Chapter 8

···

Make-Your-Own Mixes

PANCAKE MIXES, CAKE MIXES, BROWNIE MIXES,
AND MORE

For the longest time, I didn't understand baking mixes. I mean, why pay a premium for a box with just a few ingredients in it when you could just as easily buy those few ingredients and make something from scratch? There's certainly no shortage of basic recipes out there. And baking from a mix doesn't save nearly as much time as it pretends to. Does it?

I knew there was something I had overlooked, some real value-added that I had ignored. I was aware that mine was a lone voice among a chorus of people singing another tune.

Then I got it.

It's not just "time savings" after all. Time savings are nice, and we all instinctively gravitate toward what seems to be the shortest distance to our destination. But that's not the real lure of a boxed baking mix. It's the guaranteed success.

When baking mixes were first introduced, they were even simpler to prepare. But they didn't sell as well as had been anticipated. So they took a bit of the magic out of the mixes by giving the home cook more steps to follow: Add a couple of eggs, some oil, plus the water. And the mixes soared in popularity, and haven't slowed down much since. They hold the key to home-baked goodness, without fear of failure. Guaranteed success is what we want—what we need—at 9:30 p.m. the night before the school bake sale that your son forgot to tell you about until that afternoon. Oops—sorry, Mom! We don't have time to test out a new recipe. We can't get it wrong before getting it right. Our lives are busy. We need a sure thing.

Now that I really and truly do get it, I'd like to introduce you to the concept of making your own baking mixes. If you weigh your ingredients with a simple digital kitchen scale, you can ensure accuracy similar to what you're used to from a box. I have a basic, entry-level silver Escali Primo Digital Multifunctional Scale, and it costs about $22 on Amazon.com. Some other colors are a few dollars more, if you want to go all out!

So, with scale in hand and without further ado, I bring you make-your-own mixes that you can keep on hand in your pantry for whenever the need arises. All the success, little fuss, and much less expense.

- Dairy-Free Make-Your-Own Chocolate Cake Mix
- Make-Your-Own Vanilla Cake Mix
- Dairy-Free Make-Your-Own Vanilla Cake Mix
- Make-Your-Own Pancake and Waffle Mix
- Make-Your-Own Brownie Mix
- Make-Your-Own Sugar Cookie Mix
- Make-Your-Own Butter Cookie Mix
- Make-Your-Own Mix-In Muffin Mix
- Make-Your-Own Scone Mix
- Make-Your-Own Chocolate Scone Mix
- Make-Your-Own Chocolate Chip Cookie Mix
- Make-Your-Own Double Chocolate Chip Cookie Mix
- Make-Your-Own Snickerdoodle Cookie Mix

Dairy-Free Make-Your-Own Chocolate Cake Mix

MAKES ENOUGH MIX FOR ONE 9-INCH ROUND CAKE OR 12 CUPCAKES

Can be doubled or halved easily

....

Ever find yourself searching for a beautiful but inexpensive hostess gift to bring to a last-minute dinner invitation? Try layering the ingredients of this chocolate cake mix (or any of the other make-your-own mixes) into a 1-liter mason jar (a sheet of printer paper makes a great funnel), jotting down the wet ingredients to be added and the baking time, and tying it with a pretty ribbon. Voilà—instant gift. I do it all the time, and if the hostess isn't gluten-free, I don't even bother mentioning that the mix is. That's the beauty of making gluten-free food that tastes good, period. Not just "good, for gluten-free."

1 cup (140 g) high-quality all-purpose gluten-free flour

½ teaspoon xanthan gum (omit if your blend already contains it)

¾ cup (60 g) unsweetened natural cocoa powder

1 teaspoon baking powder

½ teaspoon baking soda

¼ teaspoon kosher salt

1 cup (200 g) sugar

1. Place all the ingredients in a large bowl and whisk well. Store in an airtight container until ready to use.

Dairy-Free Chocolate Cake or Cupcakes

Time Estimate: 5 minutes active time, 19 to 25 minutes inactive time

1 batch Dairy-Free Make-Your-Own Chocolate Cake Mix

¾ cup water, at room temperature

6 tablespoons (84 g) vegetable oil

2 extra-large eggs, at room temperature, lightly beaten

191

1. Preheat your oven to 350°F. Grease a 9-inch round cake pan or a standard 12-cup muffin tin and set it aside.

2. Place the dry cake mix in a large bowl and add the water, vegetable oil, and eggs. Mix well. Transfer to the prepared cake pan or fill the prepared muffin cups about three-quarters of the way full.

3. Bake for about 25 minutes for the cake or 19 minutes for the cupcakes, or until a toothpick inserted into the center comes out clean. Allow to cool completely in the pan.

Make-Your-Own Vanilla Cake Mix

MAKES ENOUGH MIX FOR ONE 9-INCH ROUND CAKE OR 12 CUPCAKES
Can be doubled or halved easily

....

If you've gotten this far in this cookbook and haven't made some Twinkie-Style Cupcakes (page 154), it might be time for one of our heart-to-hearts.

1½ cups (210 g) high-quality all-purpose gluten-free flour
¾ teaspoon xanthan gum (omit if your blend already contains it)
Scant ½ cup (43 g) cultured buttermilk blend powder (I use Saco brand), or
⅓ cup (43 g) whey powder
1 teaspoon baking powder
½ teaspoon baking soda
½ teaspoon kosher salt
1 cup (200 g) sugar

1. Place all the ingredients in a large bowl and whisk well. Store in an airtight container until ready to use.

Yellow Cake or Cupcakes

Time Estimate: 5 minutes active time, 19 to 25 minutes inactive time

1 batch Make-Your-Own Vanilla Cake Mix
⅔ cup water, at room temperature
8 tablespoons (112 g) butter, melted and cooled
1½ teaspoons pure vanilla extract
1 extra-large egg plus 1 extra-large egg white, at room temperature,
lightly beaten

1. Preheat your oven to 350°F. Grease a 9-inch round cake pan or a standard 12-cup muffin tin and set it aside.

193

2. Place the dry cake mix in a large bowl and add the water, butter, vanilla, egg, and egg white. Mix well.

3. Transfer to the prepared cake pan or fill the prepared muffin cups about three-quarters of the way full.

4. Bake for about 25 minutes for the cake or 19 minutes for the cupcakes, or until a toothpick inserted into the center comes out clean. Allow to cool completely in the pan.

Shoestring Savings

On a shoestring: $2.33 for mix alone

If you bought it: $4.85 for mix alone

Dairy-Free Make-Your-Own Vanilla Cake Mix

MAKES ENOUGH MIX FOR ONE 9-INCH ROUND CAKE OR 12 CUPCAKES

Can be doubled or halved easily

....

It can be pretty hard to find a boxed cake mix that's reliably gluten-free *and* dairy-free. I know that a lot of you who are gluten-free are also dairy-free, and I know how hard it can be to find everything you need for yourself and your family. We were dairy-free, too, when we first began eating gluten-free. I truly found it to be more challenging than gluten-free ever was, even in those very early days when there was little to nothing available on the market for gluten-free eating.

Rather than using soy as a substitute for dairy in this mix, I use almond flour, because I know that soy issues often go along with dairy issues. If you can have soy but can't have almonds, just substitute in an equal amount (by weight) of soy powder, and don't miss a beat.

1½ cups (210 g) high-quality all-purpose gluten-free flour

¾ teaspoon xanthan gum (omit if your blend already contains it)

6 tablespoons (43 g) finely ground almond flour

1 teaspoon baking powder

½ teaspoon baking soda

½ teaspoon kosher salt

1 cup (200 g) sugar

1. Place all the ingredients in a large bowl and whisk well. Store in an airtight container until ready to use.

Dairy-Free Yellow Cake or Cupcakes

Time Estimate: 5 minutes active time, 19 to 25 minutes inactive time

1 batch Dairy-Free Make-Your-Own Vanilla Cake Mix

⅔ cup water, at room temperature

8 tablespoons (96 g) vegetable shortening, melted and cooled

1½ teaspoons pure vanilla extract

1 extra-large egg plus 1 extra-large egg white, at room temperature,
   lightly beaten

1. Preheat your oven to 350°F. Grease a 9-inch round cake pan or a standard 12-cup muffin tin and set it aside.

2. Place the dry cake mix in a large bowl and add the water, shortening, vanilla, egg, and egg white. Mix well.

3. Transfer to the prepared cake pan or fill the prepared muffin cups about three-quarters of the way full.

4. Bake for about 25 minutes for the cake or 19 minutes for the cupcakes, or until a toothpick inserted into the center comes out clean. Allow to cool completely in the pan.

Make-Your-Own Pancake and Waffle Mix

SERVES 4 TO 6 PEOPLE

Can be doubled or halved easily

I have long made a pancake mix ahead of time, and stored it in one of my favorite OXO brand pop-top containers in my pantry. When you know you have it on hand, it's amazing how much more often you're willing to make pancakes on a Saturday morning. I really prefer pancakes without xantham gum, so if your flour blend doesn't already contain it, it's best to make the mix without it.

2 cups (280 g) high-quality all-purpose gluten-free flour

1 teaspoon baking powder

½ teaspoon baking soda

1 teaspoon kosher salt

1 to 2 tablespoons sugar, to your preference

1. Place all the ingredients in a large bowl and whisk well. Store in an airtight container until ready to use.

Pancakes and Waffles

Total Time Estimate: 20 minutes

1 batch Make-Your-Own Pancake and Waffle Mix

6 tablespoons (84 g) unsalted butter, melted and cooled

2½ cups milk, at room temperature (low-fat is fine, nonfat is not), plus more
    if necessary

2 extra-large eggs, at room temperature, lightly beaten

For Pancakes:

1. First heat your griddle surface or a large, nonstick pan and coat generously with butter or vegetable shortening.

2. Place the dry mix in a large bowl and and whisk to work out any lumps. Create a well in the center of the dry ingredients. Add the butter, milk, and eggs to the bowl of dry ingredients, blending well after each addition. Continue to beat until the batter comes together and you've worked out the lumps. Add more milk if necessary to maintain a pourable batter.

3. Ladle the pancake batter on the hot griddle surface, and allow to cook until bubbles begin to appear on the surface of the pancakes, 2 to 3 minutes. Flip and continue cooking for another 1 to 2 minutes, or until the underside is browned.

4. If the batter thickens while standing, add a bit of milk by the tablespoon to thin it. While you finish the batch, you can keep the pancakes warm in a 200°F oven on a parchment-lined baking sheet.

For Waffles:

1. Heat the waffle iron as per the waffle iron manufacturer's directions. Separate the eggs, reserving the egg whites and adding the yolks to the batter, and otherwise continue as directed for pancakes.

2. Whip the egg whites separately in a stand mixer fitted with the whisk attachment until they form stiff (but not dry) peaks. Fold the egg whites into the batter.

3. Prepare the waffles according to the waffle iron manufacturer's directions.

Shoestring Savings

On a shoestring: $1.36 for mix alone

If you bought it: $4.88 for mix alone

Make-Your-Own Brownie Mix

MAKES ENOUGH MIX FOR 16 BROWNIES
Can be doubled or halved easily

I also use this mix to make cheesecake brownies. Just layer a half recipe of the No-Bake Cheesecake (page 166) on top of the brownies once they've baked and cooled. And like many of the mixes in this chapter, these brownies can be made dairy-free as well, by using virgin coconut oil or vegetable shortening, or a combination (by weight) in place of the butter.

1 cup plus 2 tablespoons (88 g) high-quality all-purpose gluten-free flour
¼ teaspoon xanthan gum (omit if your blend already contains it)
½ teaspoon baking powder
¼ teaspoon baking soda
½ teaspoon kosher salt
⅓ cup (27 g) unsweetened natural cocoa powder
1 cup (200 g) sugar

1. Place all the ingredients in a large bowl and whisk well. Store in an airtight container until ready to use.

Brownies

Time Estimate: 5 minutes active time, 22 minutes inactive time

1 batch Make-Your-Own Brownie Mix
8 tablespoons (112 g) unsalted butter, melted and cooled
1 extra-large egg plus 1 extra-large egg yolk, at room temperature, lightly beaten
½ teaspoon pure vanilla extract

1. Preheat your oven to 350°F. Grease the bottom of a 9-inch square baking pan and line it with unbleached parchment paper that overhangs two opposite

sides of the pan. Grease the paper, and then place another, crisscrossed sheet of parchment paper on top that overhangs the other two sides. Set the pan aside.

2. Place the dry mix in a large bowl and whisk to work out any lumps. Add the unsalted butter, egg and egg yolk, and vanilla, and mix well.

3. Spread the batter evenly in the prepared pan and tap on the counter to break any trapped air bubbles. Place the pan in the center of the oven and bake for 22 to 25 minutes, or until a toothpick inserted into the center comes out with a few moist crumbs attached. Allow to cool in the pan before removing the brownies from the pan by the overhung pieces of parchment paper. Slice the brownies into sixteen squares and serve. To speed things up, place the slightly cooled pan in the freezer for about 10 minutes before slicing the brownies.

Shoestring Savings

On a shoestring: $1.28 for mix alone

If you bought it: $4.85 for mix alone

Make-Your-Own Sugar Cookie Mix

MAKES ABOUT 24 COOKIES OR TWO 9-INCH COOKIE PIECRUSTS

Can be doubled or halved easily

....

This mix can also be made dairy-free, by substituting an equal amount of vegetable shortening (by weight) in place of the butter, and soy powder (by weight) in place of the buttermilk blend powder or whey powder. The cookies will still come out quite well.

2 cups plus 2 tablespoons (298 g) high-quality all-purpose gluten-free flour

1 teaspoon xanthan gum (omit if your blend already contains it)

¾ teaspoon baking powder

½ teaspoon kosher salt

1 tablespoon (6 g) cultured buttermilk blend powder (I use Saco brand), or 2½ teaspoons (6 g) whey powder

1 cup (200 g) sugar

1. Place all the ingredients in a large bowl and whisk well. Store in an airtight container until ready to use.

Sugar Cookies

Time Estimate: 10 minutes active time, 10 minutes inactive time

1 batch Make-Your-Own Sugar Cookie Mix

8 tablespoons (112 g) unsalted butter, at room temperature

2 extra-large eggs, at room temperature, lightly beaten

1 teaspoon pure vanilla extract

1. Preheat your oven to 325°F. Line rimmed baking sheets with unbleached parchment paper and set them aside.

2. Place the dry cookie mix in a large bowl, and whisk to work out any lumps. Add the butter, eggs, and vanilla, and mix to combine well.

201

3. Roll the dough between two sheets of unbleached parchment paper until it is about ¼ inch thick. Refrigerate until firm or freeze briefly. If you do not chill the dough until firm, it will be very, very difficult to cut out shapes.

4. Cut out cookies with your preferred size and shape cookie cutter, and place about 1 inch apart on the prepared baking sheets. Bake until just beginning to brown on the underside, about 10 minutes. Allow to cool on the baking sheets until set. Transfer to a wire rack to cool completely.

VARIATION: To make cookie piecrust, prepare the cookie dough as indicated to make cookies, but press half of the dough into the bottom and up the sides of a 9-inch nonstick or greased pie plate. Bake at 350°F for about 8 minutes, or until just set. Allow to cool completely before filling.

Shoestring Savings

On a shoestring: $2.58 for mix alone

If you bought it: $7.20 for mix alone

Make-Your-Own Butter Cookie Mix

MAKES ENOUGH MIX FOR ABOUT 40 ICEBOX COOKIES
Can be doubled or halved easily

....

This mix can also be used to make spritz butter cookies, but shaping cookies with a cookie press is not for the faint of heart. It is one rare time when a nonstick baking sheet is your worst enemy, as the only way to create the shape that the cookie press promises is to keep the dough at room temperature and press it onto a very dry, entirely nongreasy baking sheet. Icebox cookies are just as pretty, don't you think?

1½ cups (210 g) high-quality all-purpose gluten-free flour
¾ teaspoon xanthan gum (omit if your blend already contains it)
½ cup plus 2 tablespoons (72 g) confectioners' sugar
¼ teaspoon kosher salt

1. Place all the ingredients in a large bowl and whisk well. Store in an airtight container until ready to use.

Icebox Butter Cookies

Time Estimate: 10 minutes active time, 25 minutes inactive time
(including chilling the dough)

1 batch Make-Your-Own Butter Cookie Mix
8 tablespoons (112 g) unsalted butter, at room temperature
2 extra-large egg yolks, at room temperature, lightly beaten
1 teaspoon pure vanilla extract
1 extra-large egg white, at room temperature, for brushing
Sugar in the Raw (or other large crystallized sugar), for dusting

1. Place the dry cookie mix in the bowl of your food processor fitted with the steel blade. Add the butter, the egg yolks, and the vanilla, and pulse after the addition of each ingredient.

2. Pulse again until the dough comes together in a ball. The dough should be smooth and a bit wet, but you should be able to handle it lightly.

3, Turn out the dough onto a piece of plastic wrap, close the wrap, and shape the dough into a cylinder about 1½ inches in diameter. Square each of the sides with a straight edge to form a rectangle, and place the log in the freezer until firm, about 15 minutes.

4. Preheat your oven to 325°F. Line rimmed baking sheets with unbleached parchment paper and set them aside.

5. Remove the log from the freezer, unwrap it, and slice crosswise into pieces about ¼ inch wide. Place the cookies on the prepared baking sheets, evenly spaced about 1 inch apart.

6. With a pastry brush, brush the tops of all of the cookies on the baking sheet with the egg white, and sprinkle with Sugar in the Raw.

7. Bake the cookies in the center of the oven, rotating the sheet once, until just beginning to turn lightly brown around the edges, about 10 minutes. Allow the cookies to cool completely on the pan before attempting to move them, or they will break.

Make-Your-Own Mix-In Muffin Mix

MAKES ENOUGH MIX FOR 12 MUFFINS
Can be doubled or halved easily

This is the only muffin base you will ever really need. I've tried this recipe both with and without the addition of ¼ cup of sour cream or plain yogurt, and there is just no question that it is more tender and moist with it. If you're not as concerned with having a tender crumb, you can omit the sour cream. But I'll never leave it out again. Some suggested mix-ins are 1 cup of dried or frozen blueberries or cranberries, 1 cup of semisweet chocolate chips, or 1 cup of chopped dried apricots. It's best to avoid any mix-ins with a very high moisture content, such as fresh strawberries, as they tend to cause the muffins to cave in on top (a sign of too much moisture).

1¾ cups (245 g) high-quality all-purpose gluten-free flour

¾ teaspoon xanthan gum (omit if your blend already contains it)

Scant ½ cup (43 g) cultured buttermilk blend powder (I use Saco brand), or ⅓
  cup (43 g) whey powder

1½ teaspoons baking powder

¼ teaspoon baking soda

¼ teaspoon kosher salt

½ cup (100 g) sugar

1. Place all the ingredients, except the add-in pieces referred to in the headnote, in a large bowl and whisk well. Store in an airtight container until ready to use.

Muffins

Time Estimate: 5 minutes active time, 18 minutes inactive time

1 batch Make-Your-Own Mix-In Muffin Mix

1 cup small frozen or dried add-in pieces, such as frozen blueberries or dried
  cranberries

¾ cup water, at room temperature

8 tablespoons (112 g) butter, melted and cooled

1 teaspoon pure vanilla extract

¼ cup (56 g) sour cream or plain yogurt, at room temperature

2 extra-large eggs, at room temperature, lightly beaten

1. Preheat your oven to 350°F. Grease or line a standard 12-cup muffin tin and set it aside.

2. Place the dry muffin mix in a large bowl and whisk well. Place your add-in pieces in a separate small bowl.

3. Transfer 1 tablespoon of the dry mix to the bowl of add-ins, toss to coat and set the bowl aside. To the bowl of dry ingredients, add the water, butter, vanilla, sour cream, and eggs. Mix well after each addition. Add the add-ins pieces and reserved dry mix, and fold into the batter carefully until evenly distributed throughout.

4. Fill the prepared muffin cups about three-quarters of the way full. Bake in the center of the oven for 18 to 22 minutes, or until a toothpick inserted into the center of a muffin comes out mostly clean, or with only a few moist crumbs attached. Allow to cool completely in the pan before serving.

Shoestring Savings

On a shoestring: $2.70 for mix alone

If you bought it: $6.95 for mix alone

Make-Your-Own Scone Mix

MAKES ENOUGH MIX FOR 8 SCONES

Can be doubled or halved easily

....

Whereas muffins are mini-cakes, scones are pastries. And like all pastries, the keys to success are to keep all of your ingredients freezing cold until they hit the heat of the oven, and to not to break up the butter into tiny pieces or your scones simply won't be as light and flaky as you expect pastry to be. If you ever find yourself wondering whether you should make the butter pieces smaller, don't! Better too big than too small. And to make these dairy-free, use vegetable shortening in place of the butter, and soy powder (by weight) in place of the buttermilk blend powder or whey powder.

2 cups (280 g) high-quality all-purpose gluten-free flour

1 teaspoon xanthan gum (omit if your blend already contains it)

Scant ½ cup (43 g) cultured buttermilk blend powder (I use Saco brand), or ⅓
    cup (43 g) whey powder

1½ teaspoons baking powder

¼ teaspoon baking soda

½ teaspoon kosher salt

2 tablespoons (24 g) sugar

1. Place all the ingredients in a large bowl and whisk well. Store in an airtight container until ready to use.

Scones

Time Estimate: 10 minutes active time, 18 minutes inactive time

1 batch Make-Your-Own Scone Mix

1 cup frozen or dried add-in pieces, such as frozen blueberries
    or dried cranberries

5 tablespoons (70 g) unsalted butter, cut into large chunks and chilled

¾ cup cold water, plus ice cubes (cubes don't count in the volume measurement)

1. Preheat your oven to 400°F. Line a rimmed baking sheet with unbleached parchment paper and set it aside.

2. Place the dry scone mix in a large bowl, and your add-in item in a separate small bowl. Transfer 1 tablespoon of the dry mix to the bowl of add-ins, toss to coat and then set the bowl aside.

3. Add the butter to the bowl of dry ingredients. Toss the butter in the dry ingredients to coat the chunks of butter. Press each chunk of butter between your thumb and forefinger to flatten. Add the add-in pieces and reserved dry mix, and mix well.

4. Create a well in the mixture and add the ice cold water. Mix just until the dough begins to come together.

5. Handling the dough as little as possible, with well-floured hands, turn the dough out onto a lightly floured piece of unbleached parchment paper, and pat into a rectangle about ½ inch thick. Cut the dough into eight triangles, or cut out eight circles with a floured biscuit cutter. Place the triangles or rounds about an inch apart on the prepared baking sheet. Brush with a bit of milk and sprinkle with a tiny bit of sugar, if you like.

6. Place the baking sheet in the freezer for about 15 minutes, or until the scones are firm and well chilled. Transfer the baking sheet to the center of the oven and bake the scones for about 18 minutes, or until they are puffed and slightly brown around the edges. Serve warm or at room temperature.

Shoestring Savings

On a shoestring: $2.88 for mix alone

If you bought it: $8.32 for mix alone

Make-Your-Own Chocolate Scone Mix

MAKES ENOUGH MIX FOR 8 SCONES

Can be doubled or halved easily

....

I like these chocolate scones best with ¾ cup semisweet chocolate chips and ½ cup dried sour cherries. If you want the dried fruit to keep from getting too chewy during baking, try soaking it in warm water for 7 or 8 minutes, then draining before adding it to the mix. Or use frozen cherries, sliced in half while still frozen, in place of dried. To make the scones dairy-free, use vegetable shortening in place of the butter, and soy powder (by weight) in place of the buttermilk blend powder or whey powder.

1¾ cup (245 g) high-quality all-purpose gluten-free flour

¾ teaspoon xanthan gum (omit if your blend already contains it)

5 tablespoons (25 g) natural unsweetened cocoa powder

Scant ½ cup (43 g) cultured buttermilk blend powder (I use Saco brand), or ⅓
    cup (43 g) whey powder

2 teaspoons baking powder

1 teaspoon baking soda

½ teaspoon kosher salt

5 tablespoons (60 g) sugar

1. Place all ingredients in a large bowl and whisk well. Store in an airtight container until ready to use.

Chocolate Scones

Time Estimate: 10 minutes active time, 18 minutes inactive time

1 batch Make-Your-Own Chocolate Scone Mix
1¼ cups frozen or dried add-in pieces
6 tablespoons (84 g) unsalted butter, cut into large chunks and chilled
¾ cup cold water, plus ice cubes (cubes don't count in the volume
    measurement)

1. Preheat your oven to 400°F. Line a rimmed baking sheet with unbleached parchment paper and set it aside.

2. Place the dry scone mix in a large bowl and whisk well. Place your add-in item in a separate small bowl. Transfer 1 tablespoon of the dry mix to the bowl of add-ins, and toss to coat.

3. Add the butter to the bowl of dry ingredients. Toss the chunks of butter in the dry ingredients to coat the butter. Press each chunk of butter between your thumb and forefinger to flatten. Add the add-in pieces and reserved dry mix, and mix well.

4. Create a well in the mixture and add the water. Mix well; the dough will begin to come together.

5. Line a rimmed baking sheet with unbleached parchment paper. Handling the dough as little as possible, with well-floured hands, turn the dough out onto a lightly floured piece of unbleached parchment paper, and pat into a rectangle about ½ inch. Cut the dough into eight triangles, or cut out eight circles with a floured biscuit cutter. Place the triangles (or circles) about an inch apart on the prepared baking sheet. Brush with a bit of milk and sprinkle with a tiny bit of sugar, if you like.

6. Place the baking sheet in the freezer for about 15 minutes, or until the scones are firm and well chilled. Transfer the baking sheet to the center of the oven and bake the scones for about 18 minutes, or until they are puffed and firm to the touch. Serve warm or at room temperature.

Make-Your-Own Chocolate Chip Cookie Mix

MAKES ENOUGH MIX FOR 2 DOZEN COOKIES

Can be doubled or halved easily

These cookies can be made dairy-free perhaps most easily of all. Simply use dairy-free chocolate chips, and substitute the same amount of vegetable shortening (by weight) in place of the butter. These are thick and chewy cookies, but they can be made larger and thinner by pressing down each ball of dough with your palm before baking. They have too little butter to be particularly crispy, though.

2¼ cups (315 g) high-quality all-purpose gluten-free flour
1 teaspoon xanthan gum (omit if your blend already contains it)
1 teaspoon baking soda
½ teaspoon kosher salt
¾ cup (164 g) packed light brown sugar
¾ cup (150 g) granulated sugar
12 ounces semisweet chocolate chips

1. Place all the ingredients, except the chips, in a large bowl and whisk well, being sure to get out as many of the lumps of brown sugar as possible. Add the chips and mix well. Store in an airtight container until ready to use.

Chocolate Chip Cookies

Time Estimate: 10 minutes active time, 20 minutes inactive time
(including chilling the dough)

1 batch Make-Your-Own Chocolate Chip Cookie Mix
8 tablespoons (112 g) unsalted butter, at room temperature
2 extra-large eggs, at room temperature, lightly beaten
1 teaspoon pure vanilla extract

1. Preheat your oven to 325°F. Line rimmed baking sheets with unbleached parchment paper and set them aside.

2. Place the dry cookie mix in a large bowl and whisk well. Add the butter, eggs, and vanilla, and mix well. Refrigerate until firm or freeze briefly.

3. Drop balls of dough about 1¼ inches in diameter about 2 inches apart on the prepared baking sheets. Place the baking sheets in the freezer until the dough is firm, about 10 minutes.

4. Once the dough has chilled, place the rimmed baking sheets in the preheated oven one at a time and bake until the cookies are just beginning to brown on the underside, about 10 minutes. Remove from the oven and allow the cookies to cool until firm on the baking sheets.

Shoestring Savings

On a shoestring: $1.35 for mix alone

If you bought it: $3.47 for mix alone

Make-Your-Own Double Chocolate Chip Cookie Mix

MAKES ENOUGH MIX FOR 2 DOZEN COOKIES

Can be doubled or halved easily

Just like the Make-Your-Own Chocolate Chip Cookie Mix (page 211), these double chocolate chip cookies can be made dairy-free. Just use dairy-free chocolate chips and substitute the same amount of vegetable shortening (by weight) in place of the butter. They are also thick and chewy, but the tiniest little bit thinner, naturally, than their more blond cousins.

2 cups (280 g) high-quality all-purpose gluten-free flour

1 teaspoon xanthan gum (omit if your blend already contains it)

⅔ cup (53 g) unsweetened natural cocoa powder

1 teaspoon baking soda

½ teaspoon kosher salt

1½ cups (300 g) sugar

12 ounces semisweet chocolate chips

1. Place all the ingredients, except the chips, in a large bowl and whisk well. Add the chips and mix well. Store in an airtight container until ready to use.

Double Chocolate Chip Cookies

Time Estimate: 10 minutes active time, 20 minutes inactive time
(including chilling the dough)

1 batch Make-Your-Own Double Chocolate Chip Cookie Mix
8 tablespoons (112 g) unsalted butter, at room temperature
2 extra-large eggs, at room temperature, lightly beaten
2 teaspoons pure vanilla extract

1. Preheat your oven to 325°F. Line rimmed baking sheets with unbleached parchment paper and set them aside.

2. Place the dry cookie mix in a large bowl and whisk well. Place the butter, eggs, and vanilla extract, and mix well. Refrigerate until firm or freeze briefly.

3. Drop balls of dough about 1¼ inches in diameter about 2 inches apart on the prepared baking sheets. Place the baking sheets in the freezer until the dough is firm, about 10 minutes.

4. Once the dough has chilled, place the rimmed baking sheets in the preheated oven one at a time and bake until the cookies are just beginning to brown on the underside, about 10 minutes. Remove from the oven and allow the cookies to cool until firm on the baking sheets.

Make-Your-Own Snickerdoodle Cookie Mix

MAKES ENOUGH MIX FOR 2 DOZEN COOKIES

Can be doubled or halved easily

....

If I could do it and still be understood, I would rename these. I hadn't heard about snickerdoodles until long past childhood, so I'm not nostalgic—the name holds no meaning to me. I hear it with fresh ears. And I'm here to tell you that these cookies are so good they deserve a better name. I should also mention that they're easily made dairy-free, by using vegetable shortening (by weight) in place of the butter.

1¼ cups (175 g) high-quality all-purpose gluten-free flour

½ teaspoon xanthan gum (omit if your blend already contains it)

Dash (⅛ teaspoon) of kosher salt

¾ teaspoon ground cinnamon

½ teaspoon baking soda

1 teaspoon cream of tartar

¾ cup (150 g) sugar

1. Place all the ingredients in a large bowl and whisk well. Store in an airtight container until ready to use.

Shoestring Savings

On a shoestring: $1.58 for mix alone

If you bought it: $4.75 for mix alone

Snickerdoodles

Time Estimate: 10 minutes active time, 20 minutes inactive time (including chilling the dough)

1 batch Make-Your-Own Snickerdoodle Cookie Mix
7 tablespoons (98 g) unsalted butter, at room temperature
2 extra-large eggs, at room temperature, lightly beaten
1 teaspoon pure vanilla extract
2½ teaspoons ground cinnamon
4 tablespoons sugar

1. Place the dry cookie mix in a large bowl and whisk well. Add the butter, eggs, and vanilla, and mix well.

2. Separate the dough into two portions, wrap each tightly in plastic wrap, and freeze until firm, about 10 minutes.

3. Preheat your oven to 325°F. Line rimmed baking sheets with unbleached parchment paper and set them aside.

4. Slice each portion of dough into twenty-one pieces of roughly equal size, for a total of forty-two pieces. Roll each piece of dough between your palms until it forms a ball, and then continue rolling to flatten the ball a bit into a disk.

5. In a flat bowl, combine the ground cinnamon and sugar. Toss each disk in the cinnamon-sugar until it is well coated. Place the balls of dough about 2 inches apart on the prepared baking sheets, and place in the freezer for about 10 minutes, until firm again.

6. One at a time, place the rimmed baking sheets in the center of the preheated oven and bake for 10 to 12 minutes, or until the cookies are either pale but flat, 10 minutes, or a tiny bit crisped around the edges, 12 minutes. Allow to cool on the baking sheets for about 10 minutes, until firm, then transfer to a wire rack to cool completely.

METRIC CONVERSIONS

....

The recipes in this book have not been tested with metric measurements, so some variations might occur.

Remember that the weight of dry ingredients varies according to the volume or density factor: 1 cup of flour weighs far less than 1 cup of sugar, and 1 tablespoon doesn't necessarily hold 3 teaspoons.

General Formula for Metric Conversion

Ounces to grams	ounces × 28.35 = grams
Grams to ounces	grams × 0.035 = ounces
Pounds to grams	pounds × 453.5 = grams
Pounds to kilograms	pounds × 0.45 = kilograms
Cups to liters	cups × 0.24 = liters
Fahrenheit to Celsius	(°F − 32) × 5 ÷ 9 = °C
Celsius to Fahrenheit	(°C × 9) ÷ 5 + 32 = °F

Volume (Liquid) Measurements

1 teaspoon = ⅙ fluid ounce = 5 milliliters
1 tablespoon = ½ fluid ounce = 15 milliliters
2 tablespoons = 1 fluid ounce = 30 milliliters
¼ cup = 2 fluid ounces = 60 milliliters
⅓ cup = 2⅔ fluid ounces = 79 milliliters
½ cup = 4 fluid ounces = 118 milliliters
1 cup or ½ pint = 8 fluid ounces = 250 milliliters
2 cups or 1 pint = 16 fluid ounces = 500 milliliters
4 cups or 1 quart = 32 fluid ounces = 1,000 milliliters
1 gallon = 4 liters

Volume (Dry) Measurements

¼ teaspoon = 1 milliliter

½ teaspoon = 2 milliliters

¾ teaspoon = 4 milliliters

1 teaspoon = 5 milliliters

1 tablespoon = 15 milliliters

¼ cup = 59 milliliters

⅓ cup = 79 milliliters

½ cup = 118 milliliters

⅔ cup = 158 milliliters

¾ cup = 177 milliliters

1 cup = 225 milliliters

4 cups or 1 quart = 1 liter

½ gallon = 2 liters

1 gallon = 4 liters

Weight (Mass) Measurements

1 ounce = 30 grams

2 ounces = 55 grams

3 ounces = 85 grams

4 ounces = ¼ pound = 125 grams

8 ounces = ½ pound = 240 grams

12 ounces = ¾ pound = 375 grams

16 ounces = 1 pound = 454 grams

Linear Measurements

½ in = 1½ cm

1 inch = 2½ cm

6 inches = 15 cm

8 inches = 20 cm

10 inches = 25 cm

12 inches = 30 cm

20 inches = 50 cm

Oven Temperature Equivalents, Fahrenheit (F) and Celsius (C)

100°F = 38°C

200°F = 95°C

250°F = 120°C

300°F = 150°C

350°F = 180°C

400°F = 205°C

450°F = 230° C

ACKNOWLEDGMENTS

Saying "thank you," especially to people who aren't obligated to reciprocate, is one of my favorite things to do. And not just because it makes me feel virtuous. I try to teach my children to have an attitude for gratitude, because it makes the world a better place. Let's see if I can put my money where my mouth is.

To my husband, who this time goes first: thank you. Thank you for your steadfast belief that these cookbooks are, simply, important. You may be a man of few words, but your tireless promotion of this book and its predecessor speaks volumes. Thank you, also, for having a real job.

To my three children, thank you for bearing the mantle of your mixed emotions about my being a cookbook author. Part of each of you is thrilled that your mom is a published author, and that I work from home now. And part of each of you just wants me to leave the kitchen behind, and come shoot some hoops with you whenever you're free. Also, thank you for *trying* not to ask "whatcha making?" all day long.

To my agent, Brandi Bowles. Thank you for plucking me out of obscurity, for not pulling any punches, and for being such a trusted voice in a world that can be, by turns, both confusing and confounding. I don't know how I'd do this without you. Please don't ever make me find out.

To my erstwhile editor, Katie McHugh. You may very well have ruined me for any and all other editors until the end of time. Your integrity, wisdom, and diligence are unequaled and well-known, but perhaps my favorite part of working with you is your sense of humor. Who else is smart enough to know that "LOL," where appropriate, is a very important editorial note?

To my current editor, Christine Dore. Thank you for picking up where Katie left off, without breaking a sweat. You really provided a secure, soft landing, and I'm truly grateful.

To all the other professionals at Perseus Books, who graciously walked me through this entire process, yet again, since apparently I was abducted by memory-erasing aliens sometime between the publication of the first book and this one: thank you for your patience and skill.

To my blog readers: thank you for indulging me in the most important recipe laboratory and play space a recipe-writing girl could ask for. And a special thank you to those of you who buy my cookbooks. I know many of you do it as a way to say "thank you," and I want you to know that's not lost on me. You make the blog possible for everyone else. And for me. And, really, if you think about it, you make it possible for my children to have me at home with them. Actually, I'll leave it to them to decide if they *really* want to thank you for that. They'll have to get back to you in about twelve years, when they're grown.

INDEX

....

ABOUT THE AUTHOR

Nicole Hunn is the personality behind the *Gluten-Free on a Shoestring* blog, featured in the *New York Times*, the New York Daily News, and Epicurious.com, and is the author of *Gluten-Free on a Shoestring: 125 Easy Recipes for Eating Well on the Cheap* (DaCapo Press, 2011). She lives with her family in Westchester County, New York. Visit her Web site at http://glutenfreeonashoestring.com.